What people
BELLY LAUGHS AND BABIES...

"It seems there is an endless supply of stories that expectant and new parents go through, and it certainly is fun to have them chronicled in such a way as you have in the book."

Peter Anthony Holder, CJAD Radio, Canada

"My daughter-in-law is five months pregnant at the present time and she has really enjoyed the book. I believe these are the kind of anecdotal episodes that a lot of young mothers really need to hear and think about."

Jimmie A. Gleason, MD
OB-GYN for thirty-five years, over 10,000 babies delivered

"The first night we had your book we had a small family dinner with my parents and sister's family. We had tears pouring down our cheeks from laughing so hard. I wholeheartedly recommend this book to all parents and parents-to-be. The stories capture the humorous essence of being a parent and help you keep a lighter perspective while on the parenting track. A little humor a day keeps the grouchies away!"

Diane Babcock and Sharon Wilcox,
Publishers, *Mother and Child Reunion*

"*Belly Laughs and Babies* is a perfect baby shower gift for first time parents, for new grandparents, even for parents on their third or fourth ride on the maternity merry-go-round. It is nice to know that there are others out there experiencing the same silly moments pregnancies seem to inspire."

Sharon Galligar Chance,
Times Record News

"Reading *Belly Laughs and Babies* makes me want to share a couple of my own parenting stories! I hope each edition is as warm and amusing as the first — and as big a success. I'm sure it will be."

Virginia McDonough,
magazine editor, mother of two

"My husband and I have enjoyed many quiet days and evenings reading your book and laughing together. The stories have been quite enlightening as we embark on our parenthood journey."

Amy Totta,
new mom-to-be

"Grandmothers, too, delight in reading *Belly Laughs and Babies*. Its rich collection bridges all generations and is a light-hearted, well-appreciated gift. I give it to all my new-grandma friends. They love it as much as I do!"

Phyllis Rick,
mother of three and proud grandma-to-be

"I happened to purchase *Belly Laughs and Babies* for a baby shower I was attending. And you know, it was so much fun, it almost stole the show! Now it's a mainstay in my baby shower and baby gift repertoire!"

Barb Goodin,
teacher and mother of two

"*Belly Laughs and Babies* is a great book. It certainly stirred fond memories. I enjoyed every minute."

Tom Gray,
father of four

"When you purchase *Belly Laughs and Babies* as a gift, you're really making two gifts, because Mary donates after-tax proceeds from the book to charitable parent and baby programs."

Joyce Rabas,
The Sun Newspaper

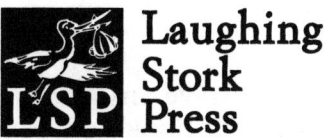

To Jim
from ESO
Christmas 1999

see p. 67

30 Jan

from CSO
Christmas 1999

see p 67

Belly Laughs and Babies

2nd Delivery

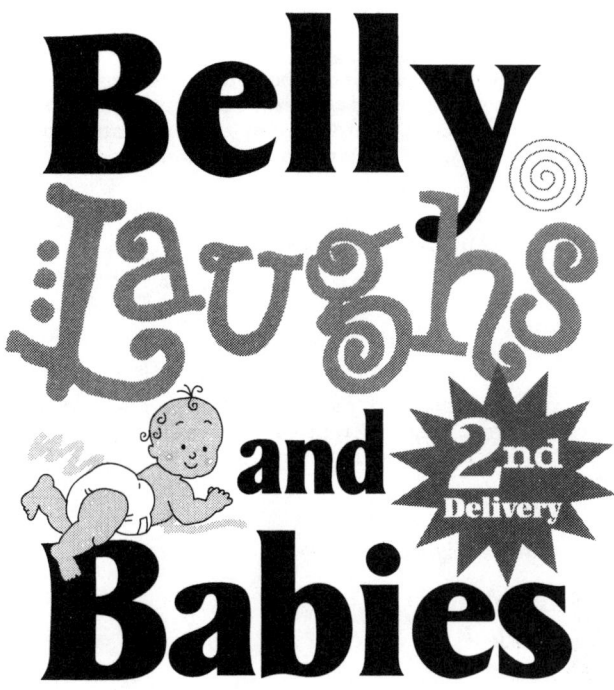

More heartwarming and humorous true-life stories from pregnancy to crazed new parenthood!

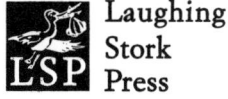

Laughing Stork Press

www.bellylaughs.com

All rights reserved. No part of this book may be reproduced or transmitted in any form or by any means, electronic or mechanical, including photocopying, recording or by any information storage and retrieval system, without written permission from the author.

Copyright ©1999 by Laughing Stork Press

Any references to registered trademarks incorporated herein are purely coincidental. These references are not made for the purpose of drawing upon the goodwill and intrinsic value of such trademarks.

A Publication of Laughing Stork Press

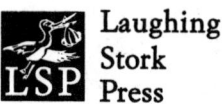
Laughing Stork Press

P.O. Box 860700 • Shawnee Mission, KS 66286

Books may be purchased for business or sales promotional use. For information please write:
Special Markets Department, Laughing Stork Press, Inc.,
P.O. Box 860700, Shawnee Mission, KS 66286.

Library of Congress Catalog Card Number 99-60916

ISBN 0-9657260-2-9

Book Design and Illustrations by Melissa Muldoon

Printed in the United States of America

*To my mother and father,
whose wonderful love, support, and sense of humor
have prepared me well for life's journey.*

*And to Randy, Adam, Zach and Hilary,
whose presence makes the journey worthwhile.*

m.s.

For my boys — Pat, Ryan, Michael and Kyle

m.m.

Table of Contents

Acknowledgements xiii
Introduction xv
Story by Art Linkletter xix

Chapter 1
Maternity Merriment

Precocious	3
Good Question	4
Equality	5
Tubby Tummy	6
Leave Of Absence	7
Daddy Knows Best	7
Now She's Gonna Know	8
33rd & 3rd	8
Skating On Thin Ice	12
Sympathy Pains	15
The Last Laugh	16
People Listen	17
So You Want To Get Pregnant	18
Is It Catching?	22
Ticketless	23
Virile Vine	25
The Day the Plumbing Backed Up ...	26
Belly Art	29
When Irish Eyes are Smilin'	31
Give Me Fifty	33

Chapter 1
Maternity Merriment (Cont'd.)

Mantra Mom 36
Sneak Peek 36
Glamor Queen 38
Sparring Partners 39
Madonna & Child 41
Can't Hardly Wait 42
A Day on the Trail 43
Big Surprises 46
A Keen Sense of Sight 48
Too Many Bonbons 49
Love the One Your With 50
My Cup Runneth Over 51
Beach Blanket Bingo 54
Stuck 56
The Seed Aisle 59
Model Mother 60
Escort? 61
Gallons of Water 62
Bountiful Harvest 63
High Hopes 63
Shower Time 64
Man's Best Friend 64
Hot, Heavy and Tired 65
Sweet Penance 67
DDD Day 70
The Name Game 72

Chapter 2
Labor Laughs

Calm in the Storm	77
De"Briefed"	77
Heavenly Entrance	78
Last Laugh	81
For the Record	83
Don't Cry For Me Argentina!	86
A Far-Flung Story	89
To the Rescue	90
Let Me Out	91
Bottoms Up	91
Table For Three	93
The Good Landlord	96
And the Award Goes To...	98
Hands Up!	101

Chapter 3
Hospital Hilarity

In the Dog House! 105
Nice Size Too 105
Baby Lotion 106
Some Other Guy 107
Shock in the Waiting Room 108
In Stitches 109
William Comes Home 110
Baby Tooth 111
Half-Baked 113
Comedy Club 114
Who Is That Masked Man? 117
In The Swim 118
Double Whammy 119
Pins And Needles 119

Chapter 4
Baby Banter

Got Milk? 123
Look, Don't Touch 124
Cowa"bungie"! 124
Boomerang Children 126
Blame it on the Baby 128
Enough is Enough! 128
All American 130

Chapter 4
Baby Banter (Cont'd.)

Milky Way	131
BYOB	133
Babies By The Schedule	137
But There's No Instruction Book	139
Lights, Camera, Action	143
A "Case" of Mistaken Identity	146
Thank God For Chocolate Chip Cookies	148
Waistline Woes	148
Missing Something?	149
Resourceful	149
Express Delivery	150
The Shape of Things to Come!	151
Sympathetic Ear	152
Full of Flavor	153
Santa's List	154
Surprise Visitor	157
Let's Pretend	158
Down in the Dumps	160
Our House	165
Little Miss Know-It-All	167
Dog Days	167
Caution! Explosive!	169

Chapter 5
Delivery Dilemmas

Born at the Slurpee Machine? 173
Coach Dad Pinch Hits 175
Cold Night, Warm Memory 182
Baby On Deck 188
Deliver Me From Due Dates 192
The Lopata Way 196
Stork 747 201

Afterward 205
Shower Invitation/Contest
Information 207
Contributor's Index 209
About the Author & Illustrator 211
Hall of Fame 213

Acknowledgments

Special thanks to our *Belly Laughs and Babies* charming illustrator, Melissa Muldoon, and her delightful family—especially baby Kyle who perfectly executed his entrance into this world with a sunny personality, much to the inspiration of us all! Book 2 was born with nary a peep or a scream. Melissa, you're the best. Breathing life into our wonderful stories is your forté! Thank you for your many, many hours of diligence. Although we bonded two years ago with *Belly Laughs and Babies 1*, it was wonderful working closely again. My love to you and the "boys"!

What a joy to work with such kind-hearted, dedicated and talented editors. My heartfelt thanks to Gail Borelli, Paula Janicke and Toni Wood for their devotion to the cause. Thank you, ladies, for your marathon editing efforts. Book two is certainly a joint endeavor! Special thanks, too, to Jennifer Heinemann, for starting us off on the right foot.

To the delightful Katy Raymond, whose sense of humor and wondrous writing ability kept Melissa and me in stitches — many, many thanks for your hours of inspired brainstorming and editing. You certainly kept the "fun" in our labor!

Many thanks to Nancy Peckham for diligently typing the thousands and thousands of words for this effort. Thank you for your kind words of encouragement, too, Nancy.

What would we do without the computer gurus to keep us chugging along the information highway trouble-free? Special thanks to Del Bethke and Ron Lewerke.

To all the parents and grandparents who have shared, and continue to share, their precious stories with us, may we continue to deserve the honor of sharing your special memories. We feel like we know you. Thank you for joining our *Belly Laughs and Babies'* family. We welcome you with open arms!

And a very sincere thank you to the following wonderful people for their support and friendship:

Lea Oelschlaeger, Maribeth Brennaman, Karen McQuiston, Lisa Shepard, Susan Summerlin, Deb Turner, Kim Stanley, Cynthia Beard, Dan Poynter, Grace Houston, Edie Pray, Allison Brown, Mary Huston, Cindi Parsons, Janice Mayberry, Betsy Vossman, Libby Brennaman, Amy Totta, Sloane Totta, Lisa Ragan, Rick Morton, Lloyd Rich, Patty Zender, Pete Heaven, Susan Dawes, Lisa Payne, Katie Baldwin, Liz Barnett, Nancy Moser, Linda Ptacek, Denny Barnett, Colin McQuillan, Andrew Vleisides, Robert Vaille, Suzette Chenard Bruha, John Decker, Dolores Decker, Jackie Randle, Doug Huston, Lisa Ferguson, Betty Sheridan, Jack Sheridan, John Bruha, Art Linkletter, and all the wonderful people involved with the original *Belly Laughs and Babies*.

And to my biggest supporters: special thanks, love and hugs to my three wonderful children, Adam, Zach, and Hilary and to my endless source of inspiration, my dear husband, Randy. Keep helping those precious babies into this world, dear. They are truly the miracles that keep us all connected with the spirit of life. Thank you, mother Clara, for your invaluable assistance and endless encouragement. You are all the best!

Special thanks, too, for the wonderful parents around the world — let's keep that sense of humor alive, each and every day. Long live parenthood fun!

Introduction

Boy, the stork is busy!

What a joy and honor to have collected nearly one thousand stork stories from parents and grandparents across America — and beyond! From Poland to Australia, new parenthood continues to sing its beautiful song and wreak havoc among the sanest of souls.

Belly up for a delightful peek into the fun-filled, anxiety-ridden, wild ride of new parenthood as the fun continues with *Belly Laughs and Babies 2*. Our new addition to the *Belly Laughs and Babies* family brings over one hundred, new, real-life stories to tickle your baby-loving heart. Push those new parenthood woes aside for a while, and indulge yourself in a little fun. You deserve it!

What fun to be awakened by a clamoring phone, announcing the impending arrival of another bundle of joy for a lucky family! Sharing a household with three lively children and a busy obstetrician/gynecologist husband serves as the inspiration for our *Belly Laughs and Babies* endeavors.

Our Stork Search continues with a flourish. I still marvel in the wonder and joy of new parenthood, and delight in the shared stories from proud parents and grandparents. From the warm comments the first *Belly Laughs and Babies* received, you delight in reading the stories as much as we love collecting them.

Imagine our excitement in receiving a letter and story from Mr. Art Linkletter! It is an honor to share one of his special fatherhood memories in this edition. As "Kids Say the Darndest Things" spreads fun across America, and beyond, Mr. Linkletter's gentle humor continues to delight millions. I truly admire and appreciate the smiles and laughter he has so generously shared.

Kids *do* say the darndest things, but as you will see, so do parents and grandparents! My sincere thanks to all the wonderful people who have shared their stork-related anecdotes and escapades. And now, it is my distinct pleasure to bring you our celebration of the lighter side of new parenthood — *Belly Laughs and Babies 2.*

Best wishes for a life-long journey of parenthood fun!

Special Thanks

To the wonderful parents, grandparents, friends, family members, and baby lovers everywhere who have shared their stork stories with *Belly Laughs and Babies*, a heartfelt THANK YOU!

Please accept our gratitude and appreciation for sharing your stork-related memories. We wish we could print every story and every individual's name, but space does not permit. However, past submissions may be selected for future *Belly Laughs and Babies* editions, so please watch for future stork deliveries.

Keep the stories coming! And thank you for your kind support of our *Belly Laughs and Babies* efforts.

Belly Laughs and Babies Celebrity Spotlight

One of my favorite childhood possessions was my well-worn paperback copy of Mr. Art Linkletter's bestseller, *Kids Say the Darndest Things*. Rereading my favorites, over and over again, I would laugh and laugh until tears were streaming down my face.

Mr. Linkletter is a remarkable man who has delighted millions with his kind-hearted sense of humor. A television and radio star for over sixty years, he continues to delight audiences with appearances on the television show, "Kids Say the Darndest Things." His most recent national bestseller is *Old Age Is Not For Sissies*.

We are thrilled to give a big *Belly Laughs and Babies* round of applause for this wonderful humanitarian. The recipient of numerous awards, including Emmys and a Grammy, Mr. Linkletter takes particular pride in one—"Grandfather of the Year."

A warm and fuzzy "thank you" to the beloved Mr. Linkletter, who contributed the following story to our *Belly Laughs and Babies* treasury. Mr. Linkletter is a treasure in himself, don't you agree?

Radio Delivery

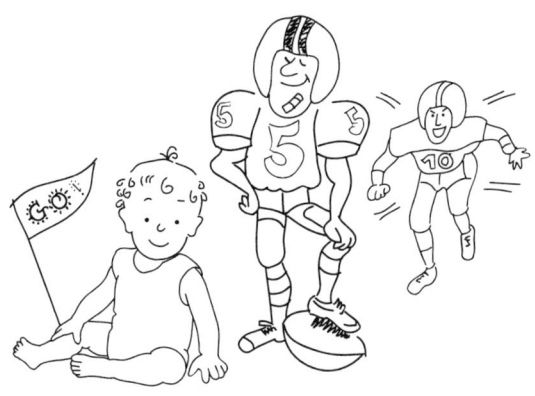

My most memorable belly laugh experience occurred during the birth of my second child. My wife was laboring in a San Francisco hospital while I was broadcasting a football game in Berkeley between the University of California and Stanford.

In the last moments before my daughter was born, my wife tells me we were both competing for the doctors' attention despite the fact I was a few miles away. The entire delivery room staff was listening to me on the radio at a tense moment in the game. In the closing moments of the contest, my wife almost gave birth to the baby by herself while frantically trying to get anyone's attention.

What made it doubly funny was half the doctors were graduates of Cal and the rest of them from Stanford, making my wife's predicament, therefore, purely incidental at the moment. The best news... Baby Linkletter came out the winner! *Mr. Art Linkletter*

Mr. Linkletter adds, "I am happy to tell you that I shared the joys and anxieties collected in your book and I congratulate you for the job you've done in recreating them. Best of luck."

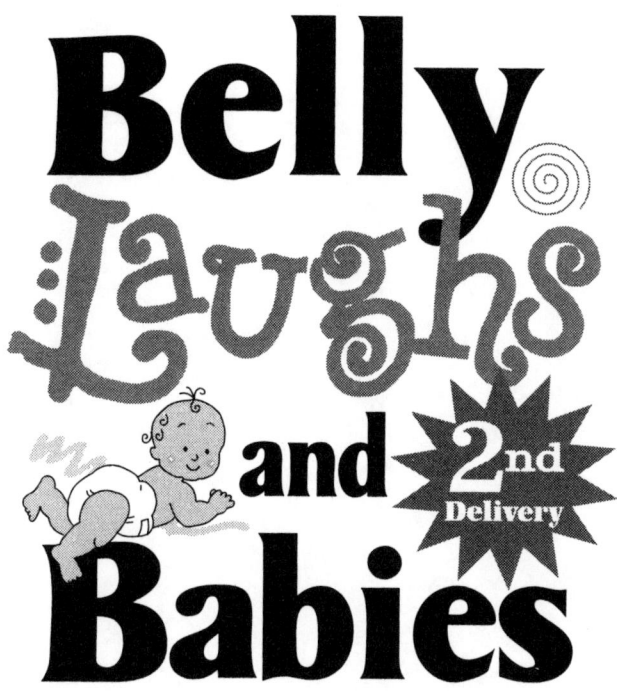

Belly Laughs and Babies

2nd Delivery

More heartwarming and humorous true-life stories from pregnancy to crazed new parenthood!

Chapter 1

Maternity Merriment

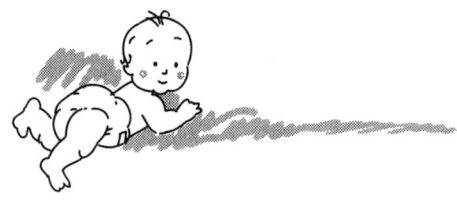

Precocious

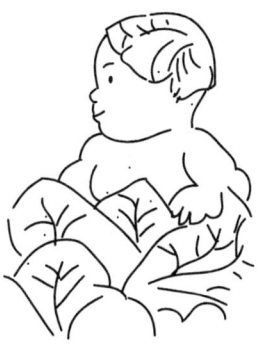

My friend Joan's first child, Christie, a delightful and precocious girl, bubbled over with questions as soon as she was old enough to put words together. Joan and her husband, Barney, determined to be totally open and forthright, answered all Christie's queries honestly and in full detail. No "found in the cabbage patch" or "the stork brought you" stories were allowed to muddy her precious little mind. No baby talk or colorful euphemisms were permitted, and parts of the body and their functions were referred to only in proper medical terms.

I was present one day when the results of their child-raising philosophy were demonstrated and soundly tested.

Joan gave a baby shower for another in our circle of friends. Her living-room was filled to capacity with happy and chattering young women. The guest of honor, Amy, in the last month of her pregnancy with a proud, round belly, lowered herself into a chair in preparation for the gift opening. At that "pregnant moment," little Christie, now a talkative, innocent four-year-old, stepped forward and planted herself in front of Amy.

In one of those sudden lulls in the conversation, the sweet, clear voice of Christie sounded: "So, who fertilized *your* egg?"

Marjorie Hopkins

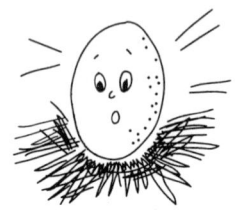

Good Question?

Being a childbirth instructor has its challenges. In the first class, I always tell the couples that no question is silly. We talk about some very embarrasing topics in childbirth classes, but we try to keep it professional. I always ask the class not to laugh when another question is asked, no matter how silly they think it is.

I believe, though, one question stood out among the rest. This is one of the reasons childbirth education classes are recommended, don't you agree?

One first-time mom-to-be inquired, *"Do I go to the hospital on my due date?"*

Next question...*please!*

Sande Park

Equality

Anything can happen (and often will) when you are a religion teacher for third-graders.

We were discussing unity in the church and how it includes people from different cultures, races and walks of life. I told the students that although we are all equal in God's eyes, some individuals still have problems accepting those who are different from themselves. We talked about racism and they eagerly gave examples of other injustices.

After covering a lot of ground, I shared another example. "In God's eyes," I explained, "men and women are equal. But in real life, men and women aren't always treated the same. Some men feel they are better than women, just because they are men," I added.

Some students looked surprised.

One particularly bright boy shouted, "That's silly! Don't the men know that without women there wouldn't be any babies?"

Uh oh. Where was this leading us? I tried to think quickly, but another bright student piped up: "Women can't have babies all by themselves, can they Mrs. L? They need a man to have babies too!"

Oh no. Now what would I say? All eyes feasted on me for a moment. Thankfully, an astute little guy came to this conclusion:

"Yeah, that's right," he said. "Because without the man, the woman wouldn't have anyone to drive her to the hospital!"

Donna Linderer

Tubby Tummy

When I was eight-and-a-half months pregnant, my husband and I were spending the evening with some friends. Their two-year-old son, Donnie, was sitting on my lap.(Well, not really sitting. You know how two-year-olds are). As he was climbing all over me, his mom asked him to be careful.

She said, "See Sandy's tummy? There's a baby in there."

Donnie reached down, grabbed the bottom of my blouse, and looked underneath. He wanted to see that baby!

"That" baby ended up being a girl — we named her

Michelle. As Michelle neared kindergarten age, she was talking to me while I was dressing one morning. She looked at my poochy tummy (which never really went away after she was born) and said, "Mommy, I wish you would eat and eat and eat so your tummy would get bigger — then *you* could have a baby!"

Sandy Hoover

Leave of Absence

I happily shared the news of our expected baby with my fifth grade students. They were very excited and had many comments and questions. One young boy, who had siblings in college anxiously asked, "How long will you be on fraternity leave?"

Marla Crisman

Daddy Knows Best

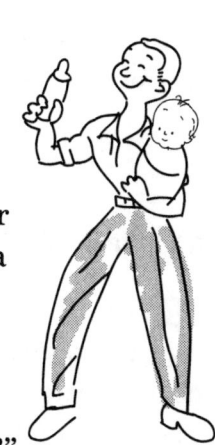

Our daughter Polly was preparing their three-and-a-half-year-old Andy for the arrival of a new baby, expected in a few months. Knowing that as a family they always talked things over before making a decision, Andy asked,

"Is this going to be OK with Daddy?"

Aurelia Pacey

Now She's Gonna Know

We had been married two-and-a-half years when I discovered I was happily pregnant! But that thrill was interrupted briefly as my husband and I picked up the phone to share the news with our parents. Suddenly my ultra-conservative "never-even-whispered-about-sex" upbringing flashed before me.

"Oh-oh," I stammered, the phone frozen midway between its cradle and my ear.

My husband sensed immediately my dilemma, and we smiled at each other and laughed. Then he dialed as I took a deep breath and sighed, "Well, she's finally gonna' know now what we've been doing!"

Wilma Davidson

33rd and 3rd

For two years we tried all the traditional methods of conceiving a baby. We tried everything (and I mean *everything*) but had no success. Finally we decided to seek an expert opinon.

After much poking, prodding and evaluating, our doctor recommended artificial insemination as the best means for my husband and me to have a baby.

At my most fertile moment, which turned out to be a Sunday at 9 a.m., we were to meet our doctor at his office to carry out the procedure. Timing was crucial. We collected my husbands goods, which we put in a sealed container in his coat pocket, raced passed the doorman, "Mornin," and out onto the street to hail a cab. We had forty-five minutes to get downtown.

"33rd and 3rd Ave.," we said to the driver simultaneously, "And we're in a rush."

"Why you in a rush?" said smiling Nagani (last name unpronounceable), cabby #2345678. "It Sunday. It beautiful day."

Now, how do you answer that? Well, Mr. Cabby, we have sperm in our pocket that needs a home? Or, my eggs are about to drop at 33rd and 3rd and we need to inseminate them before they do. Or, we're in the process of getting pregnant so step on it?!

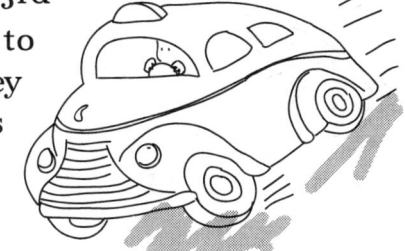

"We just are, " my husband answered.

"Yes sir," Nagani answered. "I hurry. You be there in no time."

If only Nagani knew what he was transporting. It would be great banter material for him and the other drivers on their CB radios. "Guess what #2345678 had in his back seat today?!"

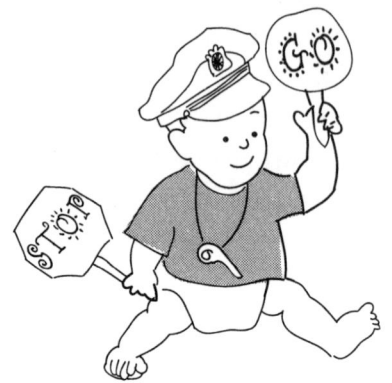

I sat back and looked at my watch, worrying about any unexpected traffic, street fairs or specimen-disturbing potholes.

I should have been worrying about waiting room gridlock because when we arrived at the doctor's office we were fifth in line! Fifth in line for parenthood at 9:30 a.m. on Sunday? Since three slow people at an ATM line is enough to make my New York feet tap and jaw clench, you can imagine what fifth in line makes me think: Who can I kill? AHHHH! But I settled for giving everyone the "how-did-you-get-here-so-early" glare as I plopped into the seat next to my husband.

For forty-five minutes we waited, watching the clock tick, tock, tick, tock, and wondering what was going on. I kept thinking about the nurse, who, two weeks before had told us, "You need to be here forty-five minutes after the sample is obtained. Then we'll inseminate you with your husband's sperm."

Well? How long would the ole' boys hold up, there in my husbands coat pocket?

Finally the nurse entered apologizing, "I'm sooo sorry," she said, "The technician overslept. We'll be starting any minute."

Overslept? Students oversleep. Sperm-Technicians do not oversleep! Did someone out there not want me to get pregnant?

But the nurse kept her word and thanks to her line-management skills, I was soon on a gurney. My eyes stared intently into bright lights. My hand held my husband's hand while a sleepy sperm-technician went to work.

Nine months later I had reason for thanks. Carly Rose was born — a six-pound, eleven-ounce naturally delivered little girl. I've been cradling her ever since, saying, "Thank you sleepy technician. Thank you nurse. Thank you Cabby 2345678."

Julie Mazer

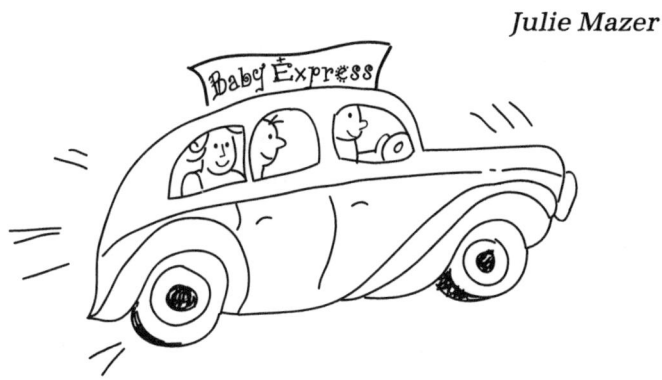

Skating on Thin Ice

There are seven couples in our childbirth preparation class. Our instructor, who also teaches aerobics for post-natal mothers, is the only woman there who can tuck in a shirt. She tells us, smiling as if modeling for a toothpaste ad, that this class is fun and we'll make lots of new friends while learning something. We look at one another across the room and then at our feet like seventh graders at a dance.

Our instructor is not discouraged. She tells us, "Before you warm up, maybe you need an ice breaker!" She laughs. We don't get it until she holds up three trays of ice. She tells us we are going to simulate labor and test our ability to handle discomfort. "She means pain," I whisper to your father, who smiles.

She dims the lights and passes out three ice cubes on a paper towel to each of the couples. I am to hold the ice in my fist, without the paper towel, for three minutes. Your father is supposed to sit behind me, rubbing my shoulders and my neck while whispering encouragement. I am not, under any circumstances, to drop the ice.

She sets an egg timer and says cheerfully, "Your first contraction is beginning! Breathe and squeeze the ice," I grip the ice in my palm and take a deep breath. For a few seconds it feels good, like cool Jell-O between my fingers. But then my hand numbs and I feel the ice seep into my vein and spread up my arm. Your 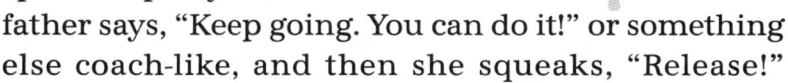 father says, "Keep going. You can do it!" or something else coach-like, and then she squeaks, "Release!"

Before the water can drip on the floor, she says, "Again!" I squeeze my hand as tight as my bladder in a long restroom line. After a few seconds, she says, "Keep going! This is a long one!" Your father says, "Come on...it's OK, you can do it" and other things that make me feel like a puppy being house-trained through positive reinforcement. After awhile she says, "Hold it one minute more!" I say, "This is stupid," and drop the ice on the floor.

Uh oh. Your father is appalled, as he always is when I'm not a joiner. "Pick it up," he hisses. "She'll see you!" I roll my eyes and say, "Fine, she can give me detention." I let the ice melt into the carpet while your father tries to kick it under my chair with his foot. He sighs.

Time is up and our instructor tells us to switch places. "Let's have the coaches feel what we're going through," she says, winking at the moms. I roll my eyes again. The discomfort of holding one measly melting ice cube is not going to compete with the pain of a full blown labor contraction! Even I, a person who's never had a child, know that.

Your father picks up the ice and sucks in a breath.

He is ready when she chirps, "Begin, coaches!" I am sitting behind him now and rub his shoulders half-heartedly. She tells us, "Remember, moms, the role of a coach is crucial!" I try to say, "You can do it," but the words get stuck in my throat. I feel like an idiot.

Your father doesn't need my encouragement. He is gripping the ice; the water is leaking onto the floor. His breathing is slow and deep. "Doesn't it hurt?" I ask him. He nods. "Just let it go," I tell him." It's stupid." He shakes his head no. The instructor peeps up, " What do you think, moms, another two minutes?" Some of the moms whoop and clap while the coaches groan. Your father is silent, his fist of ice, steady and still.

When time is up, your father is one of the only coaches in the room with a wet hand. The rest have dropped their ice. I can't help it... I am kind of impressed. As I watch him rubbing his hand, I realize this is one of the reasons that I love him, that I chose him to be my partner, your father. He is the kind of guy who sticks. When things get tough, when love turns to ice, when I want to run and let what we have seep out of my fingers, to take the easy road, to have a day in the sun–he waits through the winter for the thaw. He waits for the spring. And he does it quietly, without complaining, knowing it will come. Knowing he can wait, knowing that everything that is frozen will melt...before time begins or ends.

This is your father. Aren't we lucky?

Laurie Rachkus Uttich

Sympathy Pains

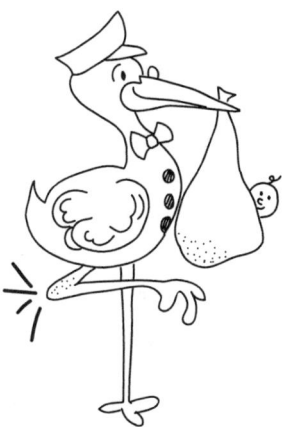

Being a first time mother, the new aches and pains of child bearing increased with each passing month and caused me great concern. I relayed each new ailment to my doctor, a man who had been delivering babies for over thirty years. Sometimes he wasn't the most sympathetic person in the world and his common response was "Yeah, that will happen," never taking his eyes off my medical chart.

In my last trimester, I became quite concerned because I developed a tingling numbness in my right leg. I mentioned this new condition to my doctor and was very surprised when he looked at me with eyes and mouth wide open. He started asking me questions. "Does it come and go, does it feel like it's on fire sometimes, does it move to different areas?" I answered "Yes!" to each question, thinking finally I had something really serious to be concerned about.

Much to my surprise, my doctor said in a sympathetic tone, "Yeah, that happens to me sometimes too. It's a pinched nerve." Whereby he finished up the exam and left the room.

Cheryl Murphy

The Last Laugh

On April 1, 1954, I decided to play an April Fool joke on two of my close friends. I telephoned Joyce and, without actually lying, gave her the impression that Bev was pregnant. Then I called Bev and hinted the same erroneous information about Joyce.

I urged Bev to call Joyce right away to cheer her up. Since Joyce already had three children with two still in diapers, I laid it on thick that she was sure to be down in the dumps. The pill was not available at the time so family planning was chancy at best.

I hung up and giggled to myself as I imagined the conversation between the two. After some time went by without a return call from either of them, I became worried that my joke would not be funny at all if it went too far.

I dialed Bev's number. She said that Joyce's line was busy, but Bev's husband had called from work so she told him the news. He had said he couldn't wait to tell his co-workers so they could all kid Clarence.

"Oh, no," I groaned. "It was a joke. April Fools, you know. Please call him back right away and tell him it's not true. And—uh—I—uh sort of made Joyce think you were p.g., too. I didn't really lie, you know, I just thought it would be funny when you both thought—"

Bev's voice exploded in my ear. "You told her I was pregnant! How could you? She's probably spreading it all over town by now. Some friend you are!" She hung up.

I felt terrible. How could I make amends? The phone rang. Glumly I picked up the receiver and two voices yelled in my ear, "April Fool!" My two friends laughed raucously. Then Bev explained that Joyce had run over to her house instead of phoning. When they realized I had tricked them, they decided to make me sweat a little.

We have laughed about it many times since, especially after I learned that the last laugh was on me. Our third son was born December 31, 1954, exactly nine months later.

Grace Houston

People Listen

One day near the end of my second pregnancy, my morning league bowling team finished early, collected children from the nursery, and settled at a table in the bowling alley's lunch area. We were shouting to be heard over the noise of balls hitting pins. Then, just as the last bowler finished and an uncharacteristic silence descended, my five-year-old daughter asked in a loud voice, "Mom, I know how the baby gets out. But how does it get in there?"

Everyone froze in a silent pose. Other bowlers, waitresses, even the mailman sitting at the lunch counter, cocked their heads toward our table. I froze too, stunned that everyone was waiting for my answer.

An E.F. Hutton commercial could not have done it better.

Mary-Lane Kamberg

So You Want To Get Pregnant

Before you commit pregnancy, read this. I have advice and information for you beyond the old wives' tales you've heard.

One of the tale tellers is your mom, who is hoping for a grandchild. Her friends flip open their Gramma's Brag Books and gloat. She wants her own Gramma's Brag Book.

Being prim and prudish, tale tellers don't tell you what happens to your sex life once you decide to have a baby. I admit that sex will become purposeful and joyful, a celebration of love with the intent of procreation — for about six weeks. After that, sex will not be initiated with passion. It will become a chore, like cleaning out the garage. Besides that, after your period comes and goes, both you and your husband will begin to feel like failures. Each will believe he/she failed to select a fertile mate.

To complicate it, you can research choosing the sex of your child. Sex will lose its passion after you discover the various and unique ways of making a boy or a girl.

If months go by and nothing happens, consider yourself blessed and get on with your career. Forget about fertility clinics. If you are curious, sit in a fertility clinic's parking lot. You'll see Jaguar, Lexus, BMW, Infinity and other luxury automobiles that cost as much as your two bedroom condo. Fertility doctors get rich. This is the primary purpose of fertility clinics.

Before you throw away those birth control pills, look at your husband carefully. If he doesn't have a college education, get him one. This is to ensure his income. He should be making enough money to send the kids to good colleges and buy homes for your grown children so you can evict them from your house at the appropriate time without guilt. It would be best if he chooses medical school and becomes a fertility doctor.

Take a look at your house. A home requires one

more bedroom than you have children – and a master bedroom, which needs to be on the opposite end of the house as the children's rooms. You will also need a family room, a recreation room, a big back yard, three bathrooms, a basement, and a four-car garage for large toys. Just a note: No matter what the size of your garage, your cars will still sit outside in the winter because the toys take on a life of their own and multiply when you are asleep at night!

If, and when, you and your husband have the education, income, and home, you may think it's time to get pregnant. Let's say that all has gone well and you've missed your period by six hours. Don't rush off and buy a home pregnancy test yet. Don't tell your husband, either. It's a popular thing now to gather 'round the ol' home pregnancy test, but you'll still have to see a doctor to confirm it.

Rather than going through all that prematurely, give yourself a few good weeks of being late. In the meantime take full advantage of the fact that you are eating for two now. Find out all the do's and don'ts of the first trimester from the pregnancy books you've already accumulated. If you don't have any yet, use these few weeks to buy some. (You should have read about what's going to happen to your body before you inflicted pregnancy on it.) You can find first trimester, edema, hemorrhoids, and other exciting new words in these books. Videos are also available to instruct you on pregnancy-speak. Get these for your husband.

Let's say your pregnancy test is positive. Hooray, hooray, whatever. Now go home and throw out all the size six, eight and ten clothing you own. You will never fit into these again and you'll be happy you have the extra space for the tarp-sized dresses you'll need later.

But don't get depressed about this. There is something wonderful happening to your body. If you never had them before, you will get them now. Big Breasts. During the first month or so of pregnancy they grow and grow. My advice is to do something fun. You will have a nice glow to your skin, and you'll be happy and excited about this new life inside you. With a buxom bosom to match, you will look terrific. (Keep in mind that I am talking about your first pregnancy and only your first pregnancy.)

This is the best opportunity in your life for a photo shoot. Put on the skimpiest bikini you can find, put on way-too-much make-up, fluff up your hair and find the camera. You might have developed a pot belly, but from the middle of the chest up you can give those babes from Baywatch a run for their money. Have your husband take some torso and head shots of you in various sultry poses. Think about something sensuous like double-fudge brownies. While smiling, say "window" or just " -dow" since that places your lips into a provocative purse. If you have a pleasing derriere, lie on your stomach on a soft-cushioned sofa. Your little belly will be camouflaged. Turn your torso toward the camera so that you display an incredible amount of cleavage, smile, and say " -dow" again. Now go throw up.

Get the pictures developed right away and take them directly to your safe-deposit box. After you've gained twenty to sixty pounds, you won't want to be reminded of how great you once looked. You won't want your children to see these pictures, either. Keep them safe so that, in the very distant future, you can slip these centerfold photos between the pictures of grandchildren in your Gramma's Brag Book and with extreme pride say, "And this is what I looked like *before* I had children. "

Mary L. Hoey

Is It Catching?

One hot summer afternoon I was mowing the lawn, and my five -year-old son was following me back and forth with his toy mower. We took a break and went into the house for a drink. I poured water into a glass, took a drink and handed my son the glass. He looked at me and asked which side of the glass I drank from. "Why do you want to know?" I asked. "'Cause I sure don't want to catch what *you* have," he replied.

I was eight months pregnant.

Leslie Lauer

Ticketless

I was a career military wife. That is, I did the full twenty years. I never liked being an army wife and agreed with the saying on t-shirts sold in every army PX — "The hardest job in the army is being an army wife." I hated the forced moves and separations, not being able to establish my career and most of all being a number — not just a number, but my sponsor's number.

Usually I'm a law-abiding citizen, but I had a few run-ins with the military police. Nothing serious. There was the time when I was pregnant with the youngest. I was in my seventh month and probably as finicky as any woman in my condition gets. It was a blazing hot day in July, dry as Texas cactus, and I had still not grown accustomed to getting baked each day. The three children and I were on our way home when an MP pulled me over for allegedly speeding. I said I could not have been speeding because I had just pulled away from a stop sign and our old van was still in first gear and could not have even reached the speed limit in first gear. The MP didn't care. I again insisted I wasn't speeding. The MP wrote a ticket anyway.

"I don't want it!" I said.

"Ma'am you have to take it," Mr. MP replied.

"No, I don't want to take it and I won't take it!"

We went back and forth and by then I was crying and Mr. Mean MP didn't know what to do. He made a forceful attempt to put the ticket into my hand. But he met with my clenched fist and firm refusal. He insisted that I take the ticket.

Finally, through tears that quickly evaporated in the cruel, Texas heat, I said, "I won't take this ticket. I don't want it. Give it to my husband."

Exasperated Mr. MP probably hadn't been taught in basic training what to do with crying, pregnant women. So he followed my instructions and took the ticket to my husband's unit.

I don't know what transpired there but not long after I arrived home, my husband exploded through the door, wide-eyed and expecting to find a catastrophe.

"Hi! What's wrong?" he said.

I had composed my psyche and my huge, hot, pregnant body was lumbering about, taking care of our needs. Calmly I replied, "Nothing. Why?"

"This MP came to my unit and gave me a speeding ticket and told me what had happened. My commanding officer released me for the rest of the week and told me to go home and see about you."

"Oh."

"But, what's wrong? Are you okay?"

"I am just fine!"

My dear husband looked confused. I knew he wouldn't figure out that it was a hormonal thing.

"But what about the ticket?" I asked, nonchalantly.

"My commanding officer took care of it. He told the MP to tear it up!"

The chain of command is a marvelous thing when the hand that rocks the cradle rules the world!

Toni Pierce Webb

Virile Vine

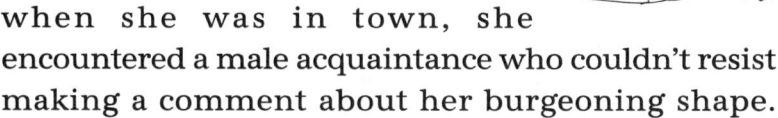

My husband tells the story of a family friend who was pregnant seventy years ago in the little town of East Lynne, Missouri. One day, when she was in town, she encountered a male acquaintance who couldn't resist making a comment about her burgeoning shape.

"Looks like you swallowed a watermelon," he said.

She replied, "If I did, I know it wasn't off of *your* vine!"

Dorothy Schindorff

The Day the Plumbing Backed Up

Functionally speaking, my body seemed to handle the pregnancy quite well. Morning sickness plagued me in the early months, but I was very fortunate not to suffer high blood pressure, water retention problems, hypoglycemia, hemorrhoids, bleeding gums, varicose veins, complexion discoloration, etc. My body plugged along very well until May 10, 1995.

It had been a long day at work when I first noticed the abdominal cramping and pressure. By 7 p.m. the pain was constant and hurt worse when I moved around. Before panicking or crying wolf, I picked up my handy-dandy pregnancy guide and went to the symptom index. I started reviewing the topics and quickly ruled out anything too serious, i.e. bleeding, fluid leakage. The symptom index put me on page sixty-four, which greeted me with the following message in big, bold letters: "CONSTIPATION."

Oh, no, not the "C" word! I had never been... you know... a day in my life. I never had to take pills or laxatives or cart a book along to pass the time. My body was turning into the body of a sixty-year-old woman! First the big bras. Then the underwear that could double as a car cover, the support hose, and now this. Would humiliations never cease?

I grabbed my purse and was off to the grocery store. I quickly bypassed the Twinkies and fudge bars and went straight for the senior citizens' aisle. With book in hand, I filled my cart with dried prunes, prune juice, shredded wheat and bran flakes. I saw the disgust in the teen-age check-out clerk's 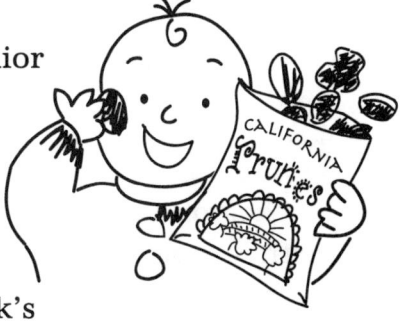 eyes, and I silently put a constipation curse on her.

I held my nose and downed a handful of the dried prunes in the parking lot. Because the book didn't say how fast they worked, I drove home quickly. I put away the groceries so my husband wouldn't have to know what was going on, or not going on. Or maybe I was just too embarassed to admit my dilemma.

I put the remaining prunes in a plain plastic bag and hid them on the top shelf of the kitchen cabinet, behind the cornstarch and brown sugar.

I knew I should have hidden them in a tampon box.

The next day my husband appeared in the living room with the clear plastic bag of you-know-what in his hands and asked, "What are these things? Did something go bad?"

Oh, the nerve of that man! He was touching my prunes! I tried to remain calm. "Jake, those are dried prunes."

He shrugged, "I didn't know you liked them." (Was he feigning ignorance, or was that a twinkle in his eye?)

"I....don't...like...them," I said through clenched teeth.

"Well, then, I'll throw them away for you," he innocently offered.

"Jake," I tried to start out nicely, "I don't eat them because I like them. Put the prunes down, walk away, (and nobody gets hurt, I wanted to add.) Just put them down and walk away."

That was all it took. Jake dropped the bag and backed away with both hands in the air, leaving me alone again with my pitiful, shriveled prunes.

Looking back, I am finally able to put all this into perspective. I guess you could say...everything came out all right in the end... at least with the baby, I mean!

Staci Breese

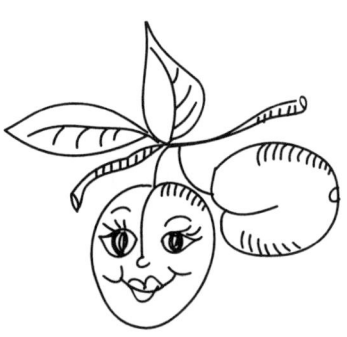

Belly Art

When I was pregnant the second time, I had a dream that strange experiments were being done to my belly. I could almost feel the wet instruments being dragged across my skin by shadowy, faceless, medical-type people, while I lay anesthetized and helpless beneath them. I woke in a bit of a panic. I had had an emergency C-section with our son, and was planning on having the natural, midwife-assisted birth with our second baby that we had planned with the first. I wanted nothing to do with hospital environments, with sharp knives and bright lights. The dream conjured up my darkest fears.

When I looked down, my panic increased. My pajama top was hiked up high on my ribs and my belly was covered with red lines. What happened? My mind touched upon all kinds of crazy things — was my belly splitting open by itself? Was the baby okay? A healthy kick reassured me on that count, but I couldn't figure out what in the world was going on. Maybe they were stretch marks? I'd never seen such bright, weeping, stretch marks in my life.

I was getting ready to call my midwife, when my three-year-old son, Arin, walked into the bedroom.

"Hi, Sweetie, how are you doing?" I asked, trying to sound calm despite my pounding heart.

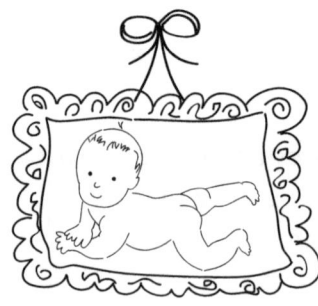

"I drew my sister when you were still asleep," he said, climbing onto the bed to give me a good-morning hug. He knew the baby was a girl even though we never had an ultrasound done.

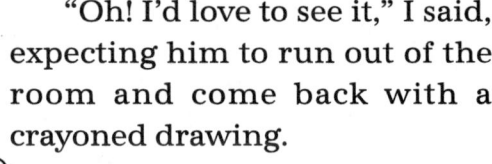

"Oh! I'd love to see it," I said, expecting him to run out of the room and come back with a crayoned drawing.

Instead, he just pointed his finger straight at my belly! I looked down and began to laugh hysterically. When I stood and looked in the mirror, there it was in full glory: a portrait Arin had drawn of his sister with red marker, right above where she actually lay curled, waiting to make her own natural and very artful entrance into the world.

It was an absolute masterpiece.

Gayle Brandeis

When Irish Eyes are Smilin'

My doctor was a dud. No smiles, no jokes, no "Hi, how are you today?" No emotion. Nothing. Zip. Zero. Nada.

Although this doctor and I had been through several troubles with this pregnancy, he acted as if he did not know me when I went in for regular prenatal exams.

I, as an expectant mother, needed him to know who I was. I wanted to think he cared about me as a patient or a person just a wee, tiny bit. I craved a positive, caring bedside manner. How could I imprint myself on the doctor's memory?

Just like "I Love Lucy's," Lucy McGillicuddy, I hatched a plan.

My March appointment just happened to fall on my favorite holiday of the entire year — St. Patrick's Day. On that grand and glorious day, I dressed in green while my husband wore a green carnation in his suit lapel. Our son, who cherished his role as the big brother, wore a green satin bow tie. Dressed up, we were going to hear the baby's heartbeat!

We waited in the examining room, giggling in anticipation of the doctor's reaction. He finally came in. He asked me some routine questions in his dreary,

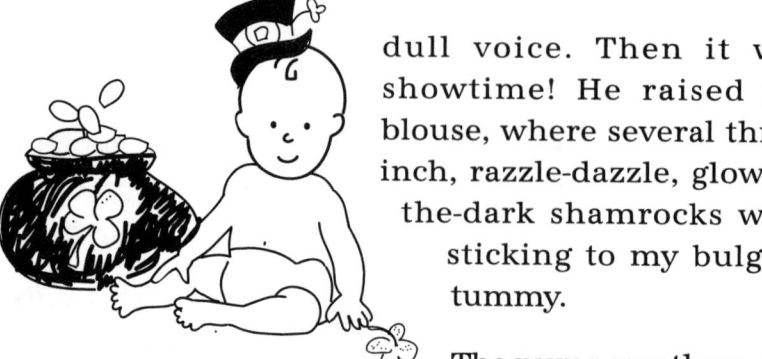

dull voice. Then it was showtime! He raised my blouse, where several three-inch, razzle-dazzle, glow-in-the-dark shamrocks were sticking to my bulging tummy.

The nurse saw them and exploded into laughter. She burst from the room to grab more nurses. They rushed in and squealed in delight. Soon the little examination room had more medical personnel than civilians. My husband grinned from ear to ear. I snickered. My son chuckled. The doctor said, "Oh."

And that was that.

About a year later I was visiting with a new friend who had recently moved to our city. She told me she heard a great story while waiting in the doctor's office.

It seems there was a young pregnant woman who had gone to the doctor for a prenatal exam on St. Patrick's Day. She threw the office in an uproar because she was wearing razzle-dazzle, glow-in-the-dark shamrock stickers all over her tummy.

I asked casually, "Who told you this story?"

"My doctor."

I said, "Oh."

And that was that.

Gilda V. Bryant

Give Me Fifty

A very extremely pregnant, overheated woman who feels as big as a garage or a Honda is told she is glowing. It's a hoax. You can try to convince yourself you are flickering like a vanilla-scented candle, but the truth is if you are anything like I was, you're not glowing, you're just plain huge.

I was looking forward to looking womanly and radiant in my first pregnancy. I thought my hair would shine and my skin would glow. I thought I would look like Julia Roberts with a refrigerator under her dress.

The truth is, I never looked worse. I was not dainty all over like some lucky women are, with just a protruding stomach to indicate pregnancy. I was huge all over. My father's sweat pants became leggings. I could not remove a ring without soap, and I could not wear any of my shoes. Every Friday morning I had doubled in size from the Monday before. There was not an inch of my body that did not expand. My nose spread from ear to ear.

I was extremely careful with what I ate in all three pregnancies, resisting the Dove bars, the laundry baskets of tortilla chips and the double cheeseburgers with everything. I ate dry toast and fruit and denied the peanut M&M's, even though they called to me like Satan to Jesus. I felt as if everywhere I went I was followed by the caption "100 times actual size."

It wouldn't have been so bad if everyone on the planet hadn't been hyper-sensitized to my weight.

The universal weight obsession starts with the monthly (and later, weekly) weigh-ins at the obstetrician's office, where a size three petite nurse has been hired solely for the purpose of humiliating mothers-to-be. As I hoist myself on the scale, Nurse Little Butt starts at zero and dramatically adds fifty-pound increments to the scale, all the while clucking and gasping in horror. She shouts my weight to the husbands in the waiting room and I smile as I say it must be an IQ test.

She writes my weight on my chart in large red letters, followed by a frowny face and six exclamation points. Ten minutes later, the doctor wants to know why my blood pressure is so high.

Never mind that I spent an extra forty-five minutes that morning, frantically scouring the closet for the clothes that weigh the least. Sometimes a sleeveless beach cover up and a pair of thongs seems appropriate...in November. I skip earrings and a watch and refuse even a sip of water or a morsel of food.

But it doesn't work. None of it does. Regardless of how little I eat and how much I hope each child would weigh at least twenty-five pounds, it doesn't matter.

The doctors who make up the pregnancy weight guidelines don't have my body. I could gain the entire twenty-four pounds (normal for the nine-month stretch) on Thanksgiving if I ate what was put in front of me. One glass of water and I could put on eight pounds. After the sixth month, my pantyhose rubbed together making that chugging sound familiar to aging waitresses in donut shops across the Midwest.

If I was feeling particularly distraught about my next weigh-in, I would drive to one of those maternity stores where they serve cookies and juice and have couches in the dressing room just in case you are overcome by the sight of your backside in a maternity bathing suit.

At the front door, a solicitous saleswoman told me how beautiful I looked. She said she couldn't believe I was so far along because I was so tiny. I liked her. I tried on a $75.00 jumper size "small." It fit. Never mind there was more fabric in this jumper than two queen size bedspreads, it was the "S" that counted.

As I tucked the American Express receipt into my purse, the saleswoman thanked me and told me to come back. She told me I was glowing. I knew it was a trick and I told her so the next ten times I came back to shop for dresses, size small.

Michele Weldon

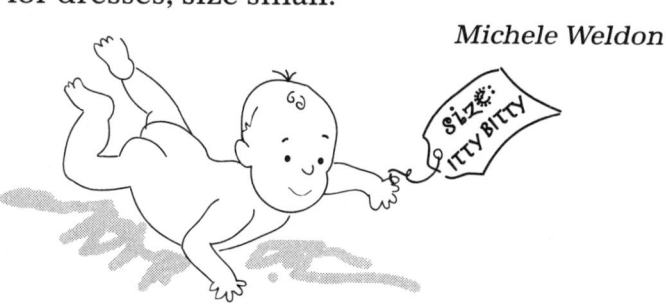

Mantra Mom

With our first child, my husband and I eagerly signed up for the mandatory Lamaze classes. However, I couldn't help but think that if breathing really could erase monumental pain, why weren't doctors using it for appendectomies? Or, better yet, prostate surgery?

We went every Tuesday for six weeks, with our floor mats and our pillows. We saw a movie on Cesarean, and I learned why they put a sheet between the mother's face and her torso. Helen, the instructor, simulated a delivery by pulling a dirt smudged, rubber, Chatty Kathy doll through a red wool hat. She told us to practice, "Hee-hee-hee-hoo" every chance we could. She asked me if I would like to think of a different breathing mantra. I responded, "Damn, damn, damn, hell."

She never called on me again.

Michele Weldon

Sneak Peek

Forty-two years ago when I was pregnant, I thought I was larger and more uncomfortable than I had been with my first child. When I asked the doctor about this, he explained that my muscles were not as tight as in my first pregnancy. He could not hear a second heartbeat, so he thought there was only a single baby.

Maternity Merriment

When I was about seven months along, I went to my former associates in the x-ray department of the hospital where I had previously worked as an x-ray technician. My friends were commenting on my size and asked if I wanted them to take an x-ray. Because of my continuing concern about how large I had become, I agreed.

I went into the dark-room by myself to develop the x-ray. As I pulled it up from the tank of solutions to determine if the film was adequately developed, I saw in front of the viewbox a film of TWO fetuses!

My husband, who was outside the closed door of the darkroom, heard me exclaim, "There's TWO!"

I then had the unusual task of presenting this information to my doctor. He was very glad to know. So were we — after the initial film shock wore off.

The babies, two boys, were born three weeks early. They weighed six-pounds one-ounce and six-pounds eight-ounces, and all was well.

Barbara J. Potts

Glamor Queen in A Dream Machine

One Saturday when I was eight-and-a-half months pregnant, my husband and I decided to spend the afternoon looking at new cars.

At the dealership, we started looking at all the family vehicles — sedans, four doors and station wagons. We climbed in and out of each model to check for leg-room and comfort.

We were just about to leave when my husband spotted a shiny red sports car — a little, low slung two-seater with a convertible top and lots of chrome. No doubt about it, the car was a beauty. He slid behind the wheel and beamed. I didn't have the heart to point out that there was absolutely no place for a baby in that vehicle. It was strictly for two people.

We were still admiring the car when a salesman stopped to tell us about all the wonderful innovations that had been built into this new model.

"Sit in it, sit in it!" the enthusiastic young salesman urged me.

"Yes, Honey, try it!" my husband said. He got out and held the door for me.

I looked doubtfully at the tiny car but carefully maneuvered myself into the seat. It was a very tight fit. I tried the wheel, looked over the dash and patted the leather seat. Yes, the car was really one to dream about.

After a minute or two, it was time to come back to the real world, and I opened the door to get out. That was when I discovered I was stuck.

For about five minutes — which seemed more like five hours — I turned this way and that way and this way trying to extricate myself from the car. The salesman became more and more flustered and finally called the office for someone to help. I began to fear I might still be stuck in the car when my due date arrived. Finally, however, someone managed to adjust the seat an inch or two and I was able to get out. Red-faced and embarrassed, my husband and I left the showroom without a backward glance. The salesman never said goodbye and we were sure that, for the first time in his life, he was very, very happy to have lost a customer.

Catherine N. Katz

Sparring Partners

My cat, Pokey, enjoyed leisurely stretching out on my belly, purring contentedly — at least she did until I was pregnant and the baby started kicking. The early fish-like movements didn't bother her, but you would have thought I'd committed a major faux pas when the baby began disturbing Pokey's sleep.

The first time my daughter gave a good healthy kick while Pokey was sleeping on my belly, Pokey just moved over a little. The second kick took her under the chin. She leaped off my belly, stared down the offender, then climbed back on. The third kick, however, was one kick too many!

Pokey swatted my belly, listened to my laughing, gave me a nasty stare and stalked away. She took the baby's vigorous movements as a personal assault. Whenever she thought I wasn't looking, she would take a swipe at my bulging belly. (And she thought I wouldn't notice?)

Yet, when my daughter was born, Pokey wouldn't let the baby out of her sight. She faced her secret sparring partner with a contented purr. No cat fights today, or ever; Pokey and baby had bonded!

Shawna Mesenbrink

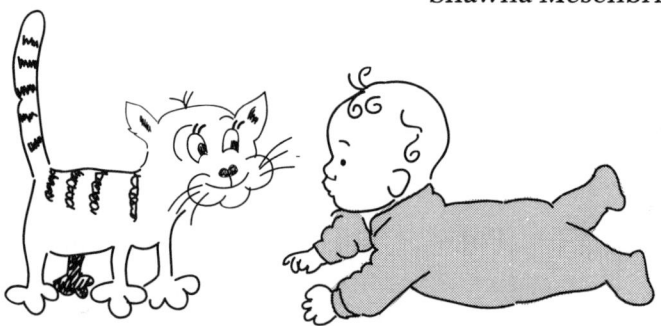

Madonna & Child

I knew that introducing the concept of pregnancy to my three-year-old daughter might be difficult, but I was pleased when Kate seemed to take the news matter-of-factly. It wasn't until several weeks later, while she was watching me get dressed, that she took note of my bulging stomach.

"Mommy, did you put your heinie on backward?" she asked.

I reassured her that this new bump was indeed still my stomach and reminded her that the baby was inside. My husband and I explained that babies come from mothers' stomachs and that she, too, had once been in my stomach. She pondered these facts with a knitted brow.

A week or so later, Kate showed a photo of our wedding to my visiting parents and announced that, since she wasn't born then, she was in Mommy's tummy. Fortunately, my parents knew otherwise, and we were able to correct this misperception before it was circulated to a larger audience.

Now we explained that babies come from God when a mommy and daddy love each other very much and want to share that love. This new explanation, of course, provoked more questions. I explained all about the abstract concepts of God and love and God's world that He shares.

When Kate told me at lunch one day that she missed God, I told her comfortingly that God is everywhere and always in her heart.

"Even here?" she asked, indicating her head.

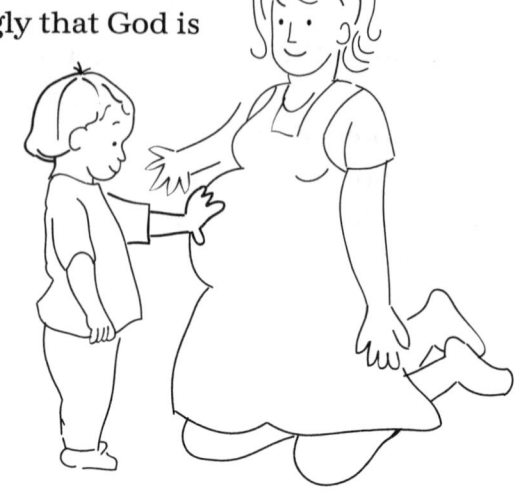

"Even there."

"And here?" She pointed at her stomach.

"There, too."

These conversations all came flooding back days later when Kate asked a visitor, "Do you want to feel God in *my* mommy's tummy?"

Noel E. Dolan

Can't Hardly Wait!

How did I guess my brand new father-in-law with-the-sense-of-humor was anxious to have grandchildren? We had spent our wedding night at a luxury hotel before leaving on our honeymoon trip. We stopped by briefly to say goodbye and he whispered in my ear, "I don't suppose I have any grandchildren on the way yet, do I?" His twinkling eyes gave him away!

Christine Morris

A Day on the Trail

It wasn't as if it was my first hike on a mountain, it was my thirteenth to be exact, on Friday the 13th. Maybe I should have taken this as an omen, but no, not me! I was ready to tackle the peaked monster regardless of some stupid superstition, and I wanted to do it before I became a mother. My stubbornness was intact.

"Hike alone? So what?" I said out loud to no one in particular. "I'm an experienced hiker and I'll do it no matter how much weight I've gained."

Just to be on the safe side, I pulled my hiking book out of my pocket and read the trail description. Part of the page was missing but that was okay. I'd go by instinct. I knew what I was doing.

Even though I found it difficult to bend down to tighten my loose boot lace, I gave it a good tug and the lace ended up in two pieces. No problem, I thought, because I always carry a spare pair.

I looked for the laces in the little pocket on the side of my pack. But they were nowhere to be found. "Not to worry," I thought. "I'll just knot them and be on my way, even though it'll feel like there are stones in my instep," I assured myself.

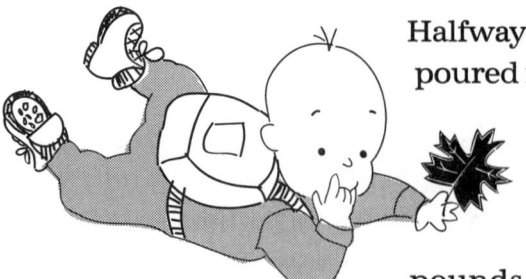

Halfway up the trail, sweat poured from my body like the waters of a leaky dam. It was hot and humid, and my extra pounds were slowing me down. But I wasn't concerned about being hot because I'd filled my insulated canteen with icy cold water before I left home.

Canteen full of water? Not anymore. Because of a neat little hole in the bottom of my canteen, it was half empty. And I thought it was sweat dripping down my thigh and leg.

"Oh well, I'll conserve," I thought.

Mother Nature has a way of providing, they say. I guess maybe that's why the sky opened up in one of those violent but short-lived thunderstorms. Sure, I was no longer thirsty, but what about my drenched body that looked like it had marinated in a rain barrel overnight? So what if my boots were full of rain water and my clothes hung heavy on my tired frame? What if I did leave my rain gear at home? I was hiking, wasn't I?

All this wild adventure made me a little tense, and of course that meant nature called, as it had been doing a lot lately. I found a tree to hide behind in order to relieve my kidneys, but a horde of deer flies must have liked the same tree. Or better still for them, they liked my exposed skin for lunch. Ouch! Ouch!

The sight of the summit gave me a surge of energy, and with a lot of huffing and puffing, I made it. Now it was time to eat.

An apple and trail mix were to be my feast, but after a few bites, I decided to take pictures and finish eating later. I carefully left the food on top of my pack and went off to photograph the spectacular scenery. It took longer than I'd anticipated.

"Back to lunch," I said. "I'm starved."

I guess the chipmunks were hungry, too. It looked as if a gang of them devoured my food. Oh, well, woodland creatures have to eat, too.

It was time to head back down the trail. The terrain didn't look the same as it had when I came up the mountain, and I realized I was lost.

"Follow the brook and you'll go in the right direction," I'd heard hikers say. Only what do you do when the brook disappears?

After about a half hour of fretting, I met two campers who knew the woods. They made me a map to the trailhead. I was on my way at last!

The map was easy to follow, and in about an hour

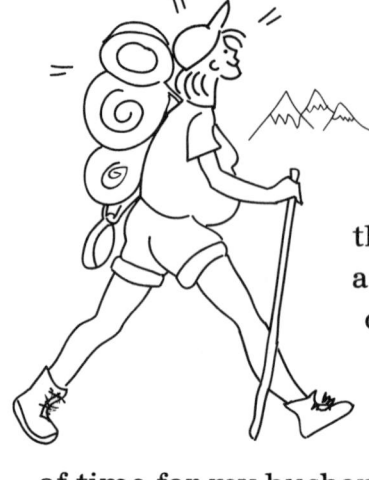

I was out of the woods. I'd hiked the monster peak and was on my way home.

By the way, did I mention that I was nine months pregnant and went into labor coming down the mountain? Luck was with me, though, because my contractions were slow and easy. I made it home in plenty of time for my husband to take me to the hospital to deliver our first, a healthy baby boy.

Jean Powis

Big Surprises Come in Small Packages

In 1985 we were preparing for the arrival of our second child. We enrolled for the "refresher" Lamaze class at our favorite hospital. When we arrived we found ourselves in a small room with a nurse and about a dozen couples we did not know. Toward the end of session one, the nurse had us all on the floor with our pillows and blankets to practice breathing. She finished the class with the classic exercise –"the tape."

I am sure you know the tape. It is the one played in total darkness. It begins with gentle music and the sound of a bubbling brook. A voice then instructs all who are listening about the difference between tense and relaxed muscles.

Again, it was totally dark. My wife, Susie, was on my left and to her left was a large burly man who looked like he was just in from a Harley Davidson rally. The voice on the tape began with, "Let's feel the difference between a tense muscle and a relaxed muscle. Begin with your toes. Tense them; now relax. Feel the difference?" It then moved to the calves, then the thighs. Each time we were told to tense the stated muscles. Then relax.

The kicker came when the voice gave the following instruction. I remember the quote exactly. "Now tense your buttocks as if holding in a bowel movement. Now relax." This time when the voice said relax, I heard a voluminous passing of gas to my left. What timing!

It was obvious that the motorcycle man had really ripped one. The entire class burst into giggles in the darkened room. The nurse kept giving us a "Shhhhhhhh!" It was no use. Suddenly we were all in junior high again. The minute Susie and I would gain composure, the couple across from us would giggle again, and we would lose it. Oh, the PAIN of trying NOT to laugh! The relaxation exercise was a total failure from that point on. I was not looking forward to the lights coming on and having to face the motorcycle man who had been the object of such laughter.

When the lights came on, the class was looking our way. I could see that a fair number suspected me! But thankfully, the nurse dismissed the class in a huff (she was NOT pleased). As Susie and I hit the hallway, I doubled over in laughter — what a relief to finally let go. I said to her, "Susie, was that incredible, I was so afraid that was going to happen to me (we had eaten chili before class), weren't you?"

To my shock she responded, "IT WAS ME!" Then I really lost it. My tiny wife had issued forth a sound that would make huge fraternity boys proud. Oh the joys of pregnancy!

Jeffrey Gall

A Keen Sense of Sight

Four-year-old Michael was excited to have a new baby brother or sister on the way. He was full of questions and observations as he watched my tummy expand while the baby grew bigger with each passing week. One day, he sagely concluded, "Mommy, when you sleep, the baby sleeps. When you eat, the baby eats. And when you open your mouth, the baby can see!"

Melissa Sykes

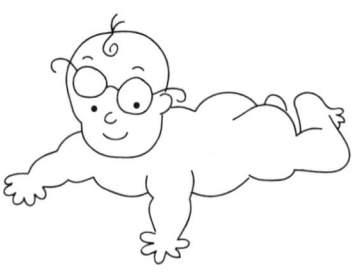

Too Many Bonbons

On a neighborhood walk with my four-year-old grandson, Tom, we passed a very pregnant young woman, Mrs. Reede, who Tom knew from his old neighborhood. Tom was not usually shy, but when Mrs. Reede and I stopped to exchange pleasantries, he became quiet and hesitant. Mrs. Reede assumed he had forgotten who she was, since Tom and his family had not been her next-door neighbors for over six months. She gave him a hug and said good-bye.

When we had walked about a half block, Tom turned around and eyed the back of Mrs. Reede and said thoughtfully, "Grandma, I know what happened to her."

I was a little astonished and somewhat embarrassed that he actually noticed the change in her appearance. The thought flashed through my mind that learning about reproduction in nursery school was definitely premature.

Before I could think of anything to say, Tom went on: "She didn't go outside to get some exercise. She just stayed home and ate *too much candy*!"

Julie Genell

Love the One You're With

My daughter was five-years-old when I was expecting my second child, and people would ask her: "Do you want a baby brother or a baby sister?" This happened everywhere we went, and I think she was beginning to think she had a choice in the matter.

When asked, she gave an adamant response: "I want a sister, and if I get a brother, I want to send him back!"

I grew tired of hearing this, so one day, I looked her straight in the eyes and said, "What if this baby gets here, takes one look at you and says that it wants a big *brother*, not a big sister? Do we get to send **you** back?

Her eyes grew big as quarters, and in a grave voice she asked, "Can you do that?"

I never answered her. I merely suggested that we take what we get and love it — boy or girl.

A few weeks later, she had a little brother in her arms, and I don't think she ever wished the baby were a girl. If she did, she wisely kept it to herself!

Donna Brown

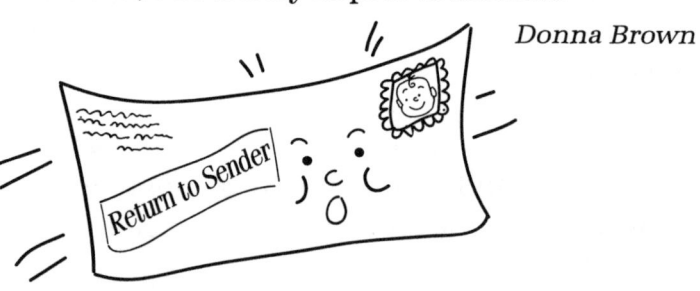

My Cup Runneth Over

It was a magnificent Monday morning in June. The air was crisp. I briskly walked through Port Authority and Time Square, trying to ignore the pungent odors of the baked cement. I continued on to work, across town and up fifteen blocks to a Madison Avenue high rise. With each measured stride, I practiced my Lamaze breathing: "Hee hee hee...haa, Hee hee hee...haa." I was a conscientious first time mother. I ate well, exercised, meditated, studied everything that had anything to do with motherhood, and would cringe at the thought of getting my unborn child near any kind of chemical substance.

The elevator doors closed as I hopped in and pushed the button for the fortieth floor. I could barely contain my excitement. Today was the day that we would find out the news: Is it twins, or a linebacker? The doctor had ordered a sonogram to get a better idea of how big this seven month fetus was.

I was working as a receptionist for a Dutch law firm. This was one of those "temporary" jobs after graduate school. It was a nice job, with great people, and fabulous benefits. My appointment was for 11:00. Rick, my husband, would pick me up, and we would lovingly walk, hand in hand, the four blocks to the lab. The orders were to drink one gallon of water before the sonogram. I have never been one to break a rule, so between the morning phone calls and faxing,

I sipped away at my pre-measured gallon of fresh spring water.

Phyllis, the office manager, had recently had a baby and had been through several sonograms. She generously shared her experience. She told me how neat it was to see the baby moving and sucking its thumb. She carefully explained the procedure so there wouldn't be any surprises. She said to be sure and take a cab.

At 10:45, Rick showed up, full of smiles, to share in this technological miracle. We said our "good-byes" to the office staff, and Phyllis hollered, "Don't forget to take a cab!"

Now Phyllis was a doll: sweet, smart, pretty, and a little neurotic. She was pretty old—at least in her mid thirties. She was raised (and spoiled) by her grandparents. Her rich uncle was a famous talent agent. He was very generous to her. Her whole life she'd had housekeepers, nannies, or someone doing everything for her. She also smoked through her entire pregnancy and had a regular diet of coffee, cola and red meat. So it was no surprise to me that she would take a cab for only four blocks.

I, on the other hand, come from hard working Midwestern, sturdy, Irish stock. My father was raised on a farm in North Dakota. I come from a long line of pioneers who had survived the potato famine, braved Indian raids, North Dakota winters, seas of locust, drought and the depression. I wasn't about to get beaten by a couple of city blocks. As we closed the office doors behind us, I turned to Rick and said, "We'll walk."

We walked to the elevator and the doors opened. As I stepped onto the elevator, my sweet adoring husband noticed that my shoelace had come untied. He knelt down to tie it for me and I hit the first floor button. As we started to descend, I felt the sudden weight of forty floors of pressure plus the weight of one, or possibly two babies, and a gallon of spring water, all pushing with immense intensity, on my cramped bladder. I fought it off, tightened, twisted, and turned every muscle I could contort, pushing the gate closed.

"Oh my gosh, I have to..." I started.

"Noooo, Honey, noooo, you can hold it!" He coached as he fumbled with my shoe laces.

Hee Hee Hee Haa...Hee Hee Hee Haa! Mind over matter, visualize...visualize...visualize what? What does one think of at a time like this? I thought of the little Dutch boy with his finger in the dike... That's good...No, that's funny! I started to laugh...That was it. No amount of exercise, or sturdy genetic make up could combat this force. One gallon of fresh spring urine came gushing to the elevator floor. There was no stopping it. It was like stopping the Niagara Falls. It seemed like it would never end...down, down 14, 13, 12, urine running down my pantyhose, tears of laughter and anguish running down my cheeks, 4, 3, 2, We only had a few seconds till the first floor doors would open. 1. Quickly Rick pushed the fortieth floor button again. We ascended, frantically planning our strategy out of this "mess." The doors opened, and I squished down the hall to the restroom, in my soaked sneakers. I cleaned up, disposed of my undergarments and my pride, changed into my spare pantyhose and headed back to the elevators.

We descended the forty stories again, in a dry elevator, this time with ease, (as the well was dry) wondering what had become of the flood. When we reached the ground floor we stepped out and heard a janitor with a bucket and a mop mutter: "Careful, d'ere's a lodda wadda in d'ere!" I raced past him, red-faced, out the front doors, held out my arm and yelled, "TAXI!"

Kathleen Kelly

Beach Blanket Bingo

There were many things I had to give up during pregnancy that I missed –that occasional glass of wine, endless cups of coffee, blue jeans and tying my own shoes.

But the thing I longed for most was restored by my ingenious husband.

Maternity Merriment

One day, in about the seventh month of my pregnancy, the two of us were relaxing on a sandy California beach. I moaned that I was feeling like a beached whale with an uneven tan. My bulging stomach would no longer allow me to flip over to sun my back.

Suddenly, my husband jumped up and began digging. Passersby gawked at him, scratched their heads and kept walking.

When the hole was complete, my husband put a beach towel over it. It looked like some kind of booby trap. I thought maybe he was trying to capture one of those bikini-clad hourglass blondes who still had a waistline.

But he helped me out of my chair and took me to the hole. He told me to get down on my knees, and he guided my bulbous middle into the hole.

It was a perfect fit. What comfort! I could actually lie on my stomach again for the first time in weeks. I could tan the backs of my legs. I could see the world from a whole new angle, and a glorious one it was.

Anonymom

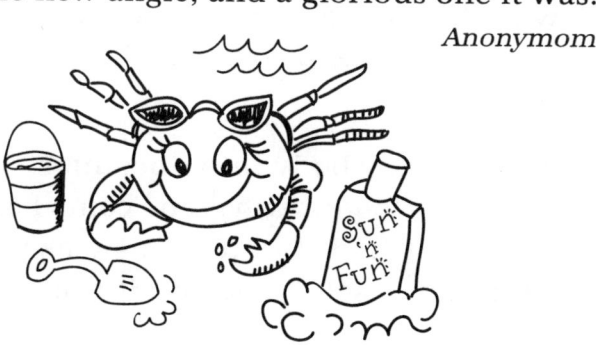

Stuck

It was the second week of December, and a fresh blanket of wet snow covered the ground. My husband informed me that he was going Christmas shopping after work and wouldn't be home until late evening.

I was eight months pregnant and was facing a long day with our two-year-old son. I decided to go on a shopping trip myself, and my son and I started getting ready for the day.

Getting ready in our small bathroom is a workout in itself. The room is so small you can sit on the toilet, wash your hands in the sink and feet in the tub all at the same time!

I took a bath and washed my hair. Then my son took a bath while I put on my makeup. Suddenly he jumped out of the tub, dripping wet, ran around me and slammed the door. Free as a bird, and naked as one, too.

Not a big deal, right? Except for the fact I was staring down at half of the door knob, still rolling on the floor. I looked up to peer through the little round hole in the door.

I twisted my body into uncomfortable positions, tried to poke toothbrushes and comb handles into the hole in the door. I even tried to break the door down, though it was solid oak. But it was no use. I was a prisoner in my own bathroom!

In the meantime, my naked, barely potty-trained son was racing through the house having a great time playing and not paying any attention to my directions.

"PUT THE BALL WITH THE STICK (yes, the doorknob) IN THE HOLE OF THE DOOR," I yelled. No luck.

While my son was gleefully running through the house, I thought of the day stretching ahead of me. No husband home until evening. The closest neighbor a mile away. I was on my own. I looked at the only way out: The bathroom window.

It was a pitifully small window, about three feet by two-and-a-half feet, that was over the middle of the tub. And it was about four-and-a-half feet off the floor. I looked at my belly, then back at the window. Oh my.

I pushed open the window, fought the screen and then the storm window. Mission accomplished, window open.

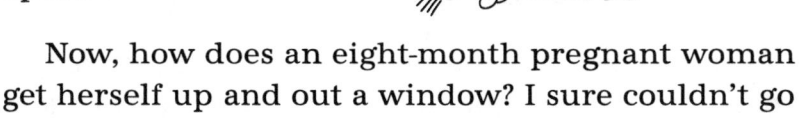

Now, how does an eight-month pregnant woman get herself up and out a window? I sure couldn't go out head first — not with this belly! Raising my legs that high, with nothing to hang on to, seemed impossible.

I turned the wastebasket upside down, hung on to the sides of the window, climbed up and sat on the window sill. My feet dangled outside, my body hung inside, and I wondered how in the world I was going to get through the window without scraping my back when I jumped to the ground. Was it even a good idea for an eight month pregnant woman to be jumping out of a window? Let alone in the dead of winter?

But I did jump, landing with bare feet in the snow. I walked to the front door of the house, then remembered: I'm locked out of the house. I never take a bath with the doors unlocked! I remembered that my car keys were in the house. And my son was too young to use the telephone to call for help.

Now I was at the front door, and my son was on the other side playing. I knocked and yelled, "IT'S MOMMY! LET ME IN!"

I heard him screaming as he ran back towards the bathroom.

Again I walked barefoot through the snow, around the house, and put my hands and face up to the bathroom window. Talking loudly, but calmly through the window, I asked him to go to the front door.

Then one more time, my feet red and cold, I stomped back through the snow and met Jared at the front door.

He was inside and I was outside. I was able, though, to talk him through the task at hand. I made it back in the house, and believe it or not, we did go shopping.

That night, you better believe my husband went right to work fixing that doorknob.

After hearing of the incident, my father-in-law was brave enough to say, "I don't want to insult you, but I'd like to have seen you go through that window. How in the world did you fit?"

That Christmas, I received the perfect gift from my father-in-law — a shiny, new doorknob!

Twyla K. Hayes

The "Seed" Aisle

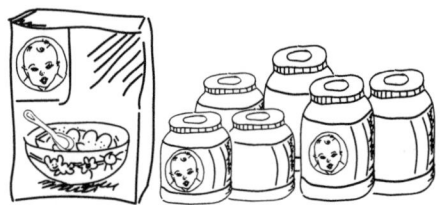

When our children were little in the '50s, we did a lot of reading about child rearing. The experts told us that parents should tell their children the facts of life when they are small, so they will accept the information more easily.

Our children were seven, four, and three when we were expecting our fourth child, so we told them the story about how babies are conceived with the planting of a seed and so forth.

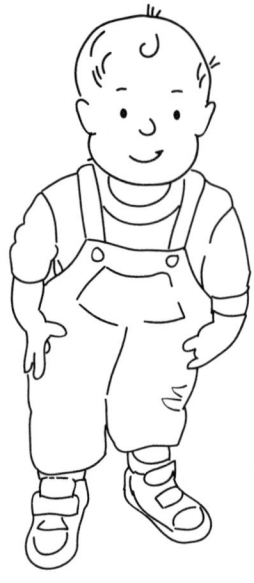

Soon after, we were all shopping in a crowded grocery store. As we happened to be traveling down the baby-food aisle, my four-year-old, to the delight of nearby shoppers, announced: *"We'll be needing this stuff soon, because daddy's been planting seeds!"*

We quit reading books on child rearing after that.

Mary Morgan

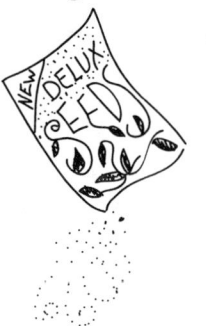

Model Mother

Many decades ago, I took my young daughter to a medical museum in Washington, D.C. One of the exhibits showed a cross section of a developing fetus in utero. It was crafted of plaster of Paris and had caught the eye of my inquisitive daughter.

As she studied the exhibit, a frown formed on her darling face and she quietly asked, "Why did they have to cut that mommy in half?"

Marjorie Hopkins

Escort?

My husband decided to wear a beeper during my ninth month of pregnancy with our first child. That way, I could reach him if I went into labor.

No one but me knew the pager number. Or so Greg thought. I did share the number with one of his co-workers when they asked.

One morning, during a staff meeting, Greg got beeped. He fled to a nearby phone to call. He was particularly flustered because the number wasn't my office number or our home phone. Greg wondered where I could be in labor.

He called the number and a woman answered: "Escort Service, may we help you?" Greg was confused, but still asked the "business" woman if his pregnant wife was there. Now, it was the woman's turn to be perplexed. Finally, it dawned on my hubby that he had been hoodwinked.

He returned to the staff meeting, red-faced. His co-workers hooted with delight. It was April 1.

Kathleen Schuckel

Gallons of Water

It was a cool, crisp April Fool's Day and I was four days away from my due date. For me, it was just one more day to be fooled by constant, irritating Braxton-Hicks contractions.

Sensing my restlessness, my husband suggested a relaxing drive to the other side of the city to look at a pre-owned swimming pool advertised for sale in the newspaper. Upon arrival, a lovely woman greeted us and escorted us around the back of her house to view the above-ground pool. The journey involved hiking up no fewer than one hundred stairs that wound maze-like through a beautifully terraced landscape.

As we neared the enormous pool, I felt a sudden gush of water. The water emanated from me and not the fabulous pool before me! My dear husband turned pale, and the gracious lady screamed.

But, more than anything, I think they were reacting to the fateful words I spoke just before my water broke: *"Gee, I wonder how many gallons of water this thing holds!"*

Susan Summerlin

Bountiful Harvest

One never knows the power of suggestion. This one caught us all by surprise.

While attending a welcoming party for a new administrator and his wife, as chairman of the OB-GYN department I extended this casual greeting: *"Welcome to the fertile fields of Kansas!"*

Their youngest child, I believe, was a teenager at the time. And guess what? I delivered their newest addition, a beautiful baby girl, approximately nine months after my innocuous welcome!

Dr. Kermit Krantz

High Hopes

Strolling down the baby aisle at the grocery store the other day, my four-year-old son casually remarked, "We don't need diapers. We don't have any babies at home."

Since I'm a couple of months pregnant, I thought it was a good opportunity to introduce the idea of a baby in a positive way, so I said, "I hope *someday* we need diapers, don't you?"

"I hope someday we need dog food or cat food," he replied.

Virginia Miller McDonough

Shower Time

Kristie and her mother were awaiting the arrival of a new baby. To prevent jealousy, Kristie's mother explained all of the unusual happenings in the household. On this particular evening, mother was invited to a baby shower.

After the usual explanations, a now bewildered Kristie asked, "How can they give the baby a shower when it hasn't been born yet?"

Wynema Colson

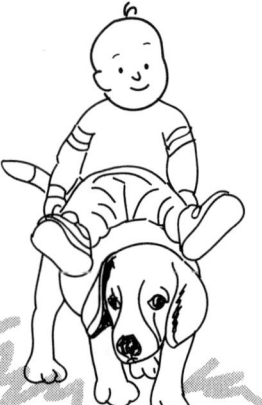

Man's Best Friend

When my husband and I were expecting our first child a few years ago, we were understandably excited when we went for the sonogram.

As the doctor pointed out the various organs and parts of the baby, we had lots of silly questions. The funniest one was when my husband, who is a veterinarian, meaning to say "limbs" asked, "Does it have all four legs?"

Lynn Welch

Hot, Heavy and Tired

Have you ever been hot and heavy and *really* tired? No, I don't mean "I feel like relaxing" tired, "Leave me alone, paaleeeease!" or "I'm ready for bed" tired. I mean bone-marrow-deep, mind-altering, muscle-numbing tired!

Once, long ago, I was that exhausted. My husband was stationed at Fort Hood, Texas, and we lived in Killeen. As usual, it was unbearably hot. And it was the first, and only, place where I experienced dust storms. You could see forever because the only vegetation was short trees, cacti, and bramble bushes. The Texas sky was endless and the merciless sun punished anyone who dared to go outside. To make matters worse, we lived in unairconditioned military housing.

Keeping me very busy were my seven-year-old and three-year-old daughters, and baby Kenya who just turned one. The fourth baby was well on the way. I was eight months pregnant and not only was my belly huge, but my entire body was swollen—from the tip of my nose to the bottom of my toes. I had gained at least sixty pounds and anyone could see my body was miserable. I'm sure the extra weight coupled with the heat(not to mention caring for three young children) were the cause of my extreme fatigue.

On this particular day, I had washed three loads of laundry before seven a.m., cooked breakfast for us, washed the dishes, made the beds, dressed the children and continued with the other endless things that mothers do on a 24-7-365 basis. After lunch, naps and picking up toys, the girls were allowed to play outside while I started dinner and continued with the 24-7-365. This was a pretty typical day.

Then to my dismay, I noticed baby Kenya was missing. I started casually looking in each room. Next I looked behind furniture and struggled to see under tables. My, my, he was playing his game of hide and seek well. Finally I placed one hand on the head boards for support and balance. Then I struggled to bend my hefty body over to look under the beds.

Still no Kenya. My mind was racing. I began to get anxious. I checked and re-checked each room again. The closets were explored. I even glanced nervously out the windows a few times. The girls were too busy playing on the swingset to be the least bit interested in what I was looking for.

In frustration I ended my search. Panic crept over me as I leaned out of the kitchen door. "Girls, girls, come here please!"

They grabbed each other's hands protectively and approached the kitchen door. This sounded serious.

"Yes, Mommy?"

"Have either of you seen Kenya? I've been looking all over for him and I can't find him *anywhere*!"

The girls' eyes got so big they looked like twin wading pools. Puzzled looks wrinkled their pretty faces. Eyeballing the situation and sensing the panic in my voice, my seven-year-old took control of the situation. She spoke calmly, yet firmly.

"*Mommy, you're holding him.*"

I glanced at my huge, pregnant hip and there sat Kenya with my fat arm wrapped around his back supporting him. He was happy as a clam. And as quiet, too!

My last child, a boy, was born a few weeks later. Everyday I pray, "God, please be merciful and don't ever let me get that hot, heavy and tired — again!"

Toni Pierce Webb

Sweet Penance

Remember when Sears had a candy counter? A *real* candy counter: no stale, overpriced expensive chocolates, but fresh and mouthwatering nonpareils, bridge mix, almond bark, citrus slices, a rainbow of naturally flavored pastel patties, peanut clusters and — Cara-Mallows. Those scrumptious, caramel-coated marshmallow pillows individually wrapped in wax paper tasted marvelous!

Almost forty years ago, I bought a large sack of Cara-Mallows after an afternoon's shopping. Eight months pregnant at the time, I was en-route to a routine checkup with my obstetrician. Unwisely, I had not taken time for lunch, so while driving to the clinic, I wolfed the entire bag of candy, licking each wrapper in sweet ecstasy.

At the doctor's office, I was weighed and required to produce a urine sample. The nurse efficiently snapped a rubber band around the jar to hold the slip of paper with my name in place and bustled to the lab room. In those days, most office nurses did their own routine lab work.

It was only a matter of minutes before an audible "AWK!" interrupted my *Good Housekeeping* story. The nurse came running out, waving a pink stick. And I was just getting to the good part.

"Get right on in there and see the Doctor!" she exclaimed. "You've got sugar!"

Sugar? I'd never had the problem before. Besides, I was feeling extremely well. Then it dawned on me! I tried to explain about the two dozen irresistible Cara-Mallows I had recently eaten, but it was to no avail. They were adamant. And I say "they," for the nurse interjected the doctor's every sentence with terrifying bits of information. It was "too dangerous to take any chances." I must be tested for diabetes.

So because of my weakness for Cara-Mallows, I fasted overnight for ten hours and returned to the clinic where

I forced down cup after cup of nauseating glucose in a daylong procedure. All this to prove I had not become diabetic.

Thankfully, the tests turned out negative. A month later I produced a healthy, beautiful baby girl. We named her Linda.

I'll have to admit that during the pregnancy, I had gained more than the acceptable twenty-five pounds. So I'll never know if Dr. Brown really thought I might be in serious trouble, or if he wanted to teach me a lesson for gorging myself on those delectable candies.

I do know I miss the candy counter at Sears. As far as I know, there are now no Cara-Mallows to be found anywhere in the universe. Were gobbling the sugar-loaded candies worth a day of torture at the doctor's office?

I'd have to say, "Yes. Oh, yes!"

Great heavens! I should have named my sweet daughter, Cara!

E. Spaulding Oliver

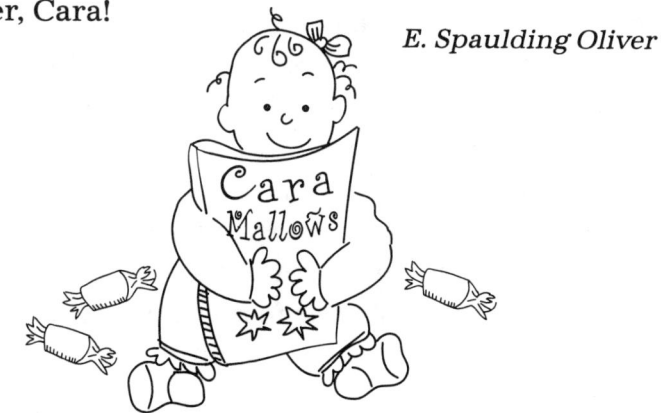

DDD Day

In October 1994, still seven months away from delivering my baby, I noticed my bras weren't big enough anymore. Oh, I squeezed in what I could and stacked the rest on top of the bra, but that creates a very unattractive look. So off I went to the department store to look for a bigger bra. Now I usually wear a 34C, so when I went shopping I kept an open mind that I would probably be wearing a D cup when I left.

I mused around the delicate pink and floral patterns for a while, until I got tired of looking for the few Ds in the cute and sexy patterns and styles. Finally, the sales lady hobbled over to me.(I say hobbled because she must have been at least seventy-five.) I explained to her my pregnancy and bra situation and she nodded knowingly. She took my hand and led me to the dark corner of the bra section. The racks were made of reinforced steel to support these huge bras that I'm sure had some other use in the heavy industry field. There were no pinks, pastels, flowers or lace. I felt the tears well up in my eyes as the whole pregnancy situation began to sink in. She sensed my shock, sadness and dismay immediately, and led me to a quiet dressing room and told me to disrobe. She suggested that perhaps it would be best if she picked what she thought to be appropriate and brought the 'equipment' to me. I wondered whether her feeble arms would have the strength to pick up the bras, but I complied with her request.

The first one that she wheeled in was this mass of beige material and hooks. I asked if it were made of corduroy, because it felt so heavy. She only chuckled. I asked if fourteen hooks were really necessary, and she smiled and nodded. I put the bra on with her assistance and then sat down to rest. To my disappointment, it fit. And short of shock absorbers, my breasts weren't going anywhere in that contraption. They didn't move an inch when I jumped or stretched. I immediately thought that I had the earthquake solution for the West Coast.

She brought in a few more styles that fit equally as well, and one even had a token piece of lace stitched across the front of the cups, for that *delicate* look. Of course, it didn't really work, unless you think putting a piece of lace on a tractor would make *it* look feminine, as well.

I was doing much better, my tears had dried and I hadn't shrieked hysterically for at least a half-an-hour...until I inadvertently saw the cup size tag that the sales lady was trying oh-so-cleverly to hide: 34DDD! That's right, 34DDD. It wasn't a typo. Did you know that they came with three Ds? I didn't. I suppose bra makers think that a 34DDD sounds better than a 34F? But it really didn't matter to me. I was already too depressed by the whole experience to care. The sweet sales lady was kind to tell me that they (my breasts) shouldn't get any larger and that by wearing this industrial equipment now, I would help retain the elasticity in my breasts so that I could wear the pretty

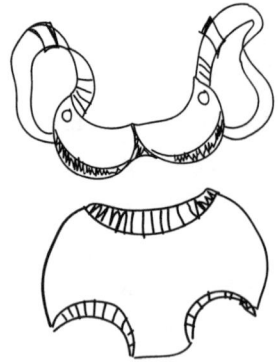

bras afterwards.

I paid for the bras (thank goodness they didn't charge by the pound or cup size) and walked out of the store wondering if they would fit into my washing machine. Or would I have to take them down to the car wash and hose them off? I also wondered if the double galvanized steel beams making up the underwires would set off metal detectors at the courthouse or airport.

It didn't occur to me that if my breasts were that large then, imagine what they would look like after delivery when my milk came in. My cup runneth over... for sure.

Staci Breese

The Name Game

I was just a ten-year-old girl awaiting another baby brother or sister. I wasn't too excited, as he/she would be the seventh brother or third sister. All in all, this new baby would be number twelve for our family! And to top it off, my parents had run out of name ideas for this new addition.

Apparently, my mother sensed the family's rather insensitivity to this new life. On a late winter day in 1961, she devised an exciting "name game." (Perhaps it was her revelation of Shirley Fontella's "Name Game" song!) The contest was open to any immediate family member. Contestants were to simply create or suggest a name for either a boy or girl. And then drop that slip of crisp paper into a black hat. Once all the entries were submitted, Mother Harvey would draw out the winning selections.

After thoughtful deliberations and careful choices, nine ballots were cast. My parents had declined to vote. In early April, the black hat was taken out of hiding and placed before Mother. Without hesitation, she pulled out two entries.

The first one was for a boy and she read it aloud with flair, "Paul Alan Harvey." Oh, the name sounded so authoritative, strong and professional. The family was expressing their affirmation. I was delighted since it was the name I entered.

To this day, I don't recall the girl's name that was selected. My baby brother, Paul Alan, was born two days before my own birthday. What a sweet blessing! However, my brother now competes with the professional commentator, Paul Harvey, for clarification. I simply tell people, *my* brother is the real Paul Harvey. (The commentator, Paul Harvey, does not use his real name—Paul Arnot.)

And since I never had my own children, it is a wonderful blessing that I actually had the thrill of naming a baby. Perhaps, the seventh son *is* a sign of God's perfection!

Marla C. Harvey

Chapter 2

Labor Laughs

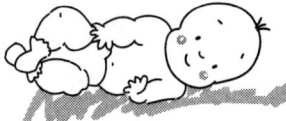

Calm in the Storm

Thirty years ago, when I was nineteen and having my first baby, there were no Lamaze classes. I knew very little about labor and having a baby. I had to ask, "How do you know when you are in labor?" I was assured that I would know.

Well, I did know. After I called my husband, Jim, home from work, we sat on the couch and started to time my contractions. Suddenly I felt a great gush of water. I jumped up and yelled, "What should I do?"

My thoughtful, wise husband stood up calmly and said, "Get off the carpet."

Nancy Myers

De"Briefed"

It was nearly midnight, and I had awakened with a weird sensation in my lower tummy. Within a minute or two, my water broke. I called for my husband to help me get dressed and collect the things we needed for the trip to the hospital.

As I donned my maternity top, I called out to him to bring me a pair of clean underwear. I could tell the excitement and stress of the moment was taking its toll on my husband's sanity. He was babbling that the prenatal classes were a huge waste, because now that it was crunch time, he couldn't remember a thing.

Well, he was right. He returned momentarily with a pair of his "tighty whitey" Jockey underwear!

Even at nine months pregnant, we weren't anywhere close to the same size.

I bewilderedly looked up at him and said, "Now what in the world am I supposed to do with those?"

Deana Ghesquierre

Heavenly Entrance

In 1958, when I was pregnant for the first time, my husband and I were living in a town far from our families. I was more than a little apprehensive about childbirth. To help myself feel more confident, I took lists of questions to my appointments with our "baby doctor," and borrowed books on pregnancy and child care from the local library. When anxiety really threatened to take over, I reminded myself that my obstetrician was the head of his department and that

I would have the baby at our Catholic hospital. I had heard that the nuns and nurses there took especially loving care of new babies and their mothers.

By the time Easter came, I was nine months and two weeks pregnant, and felt sure that at last, I was completely prepared for motherhood. All day, I rushed around the house cooking a special dinner, and folding and refolding baby clothes to make sure that everything was ready for the arrival of our baby. By evening, I was exhausted and had just dozed off in a chair when I felt some discomfort in my stomach. Gas, I thought as I relaxed again. But before long, there was another twinge and soon I had to admit that I was going into labor. My husband phoned the doctor and asked him to meet us at the hospital.

As we pulled into the dimly lit parking lot, uncertainty took over. Which door should we use? The lobby was dark and we finally decided to go in the emergency room entrance. The nurse on duty admitted me and told us to go down the hall and take one of the elevators to the fourth floor where someone would help me get ready for the labor room. But while she was talking, my mind was on contractions and all I heard was "go to the fourth floor."

When we came to an elevator, we pushed the "up" button and got in. The door opened on the fourth floor and I clung to my husband's hand as we got off and started down the hall. I was surprised by how quiet everything seemed. And the lighting was very dim. I became more puzzled with every step. As we came to the end of the hall and were about to turn the corner, a nun dressed in full habit stepped out of one of the rooms.

"How did you get in here?" she demanded, giving us a stern look.

When my husband found his voice, he tried to explain that we thought we were on the maternity floor.

"Well, this is the convent, and you are not allowed in here," the nun said crisply. But her glance softened and she smiled as she noted my expanded shape and the overnight bag. She shook her head and quickly escorted us back the way we had come.

While we waited for the elevator, the nun slowly and carefully explained that we would have to go back to the first floor, turn a corner, and get on one of the big main elevators that would take us to maternity. She piously wished us well as we descended.

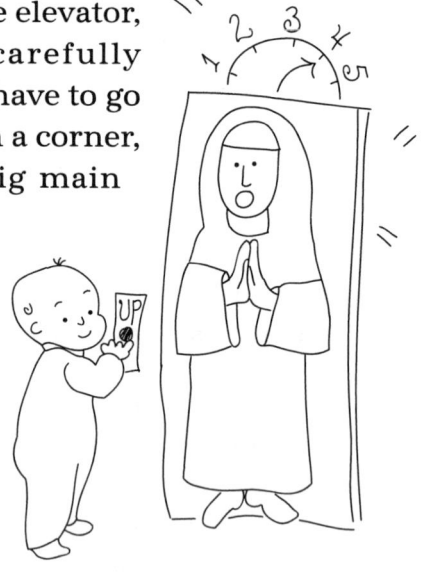

This time we followed instructions exactly and soon found ourselves in a brightly lit hallway where a smiling nurse greeted us and helped me get ready for the labor room. Everything went well and by 5:00 the next morning, we were the happy parents of a darling baby boy.

The next day, I told one of the nurses about my detour the night before and she burst out laughing. When she regained her composure, she informed me that my husband and I had somehow managed to pick the only elevator in the hospital that led directly to a part of the building used as a convent for the nuns.

My husband and I shared many laughs about our surprise trip to the convent. But when we went back to the same hospital a year later for the birth of our daughter, you can be certain that we made sure to get on the right elevator.

Cathy Katz

Last Laugh

I was working the night shift in the labor and delivery unit of a prominent university hospital. It had been one of those nights – we were seeing a lot of admissions close together. We were a couple of babies past midnight. I was the charge nurse doing initial interviews with our patients to determine their stages of labor.

Not all of our mothers-to-be were well versed in proper terminology involving labor and delivery. We always adjusted the admission dialogue to the individual. My 4 a.m. admission was a young mom-to-be experiencing rapid strong contractions. I hurried to ask her the routine questions so I could prepare her for delivery.

"Now when did your pains begin?" I asked with brisk professionalism.

"I began experiencing regular contractions at 6 p.m. last evening. They are three minutes apart," she said.

This patient, despite her youth, seemed quite comfortable with the terminology. I made a quick note on the chart as I observed the young woman's flushed face and rapid breathing. My next question was supposed to determine whether the patient was leaking amniotic fluid. A common way of asking was to say something like, "When did your bag of waters break?"

Instead, I blurted out: "Well, when did your bag of *rubbers* break?" I immediately realized my glaring error. Professionalism went out the window as I heard myself begin to laugh. I couldn't stop. Tears rolled down my face. As the young woman waited, I continued to laugh, leaning against and clutching the table where I had been recording my notes.

"Bag of *waters*...bag of *waters*, I mean," I managed

to interject, gulping for air.

After a few moments of icy silence, my young patient looked at me and replied, "My membranes are still intact. Are *yours?*"

Judith Bader Jones

For the Record

Recently, I had cause to reflect upon my blessings. Chief among them was that I bore my children in the B.C.(Before Camcorder) era.

A young pregnant friend had called to boast that her husband purchased a camcorder to record the birth of their first child.

"Isn't that the sweetest thing?" she gushed. "I just can't wait to see the whole thing on video."

I choked out the appropriate responses and hung up before I disgraced myself. Long-repressed memories of lower pelvic shaves, enemas, and vocal outbursts rushed back.

With a sigh, I re-lived my own childbirth experience on my personal VCR (Virtual Camcorder

Replacement). The images in my mind, sure enough, were as sharp as ever!

It all came back....

Two hours into labor, if I remember correctly, I promised to devote myself to good works if I survived.

My husband held up a wedding picture for me to focus on. I ripped it in shreds and snarled, "I want drugs."

"But honey," my hapless spouse said. "We decided we were going to have a *natural* birth."

I grabbed him by the neck of his hospital gown. "You *have it naturally. I want* drugs!"

After six hours, I vowed celibacy for the rest of my life.

When I swore I'd hire a hit man if he ever laid a hand on me again, my husband rang the nurse and meekly asked for pain relievers.

By the tenth straight hour of enduring pain, I rethought my strategy. Who needs a hit man? I'd do it myself. In between contractions, and sometimes during them, I fantasized about ways to finish off this man I'd promised to love and cherish.

Twelve hours into labor, I heard my husband excuse himself to have breakfast. The doctor had yet to arrive.

Alone with the nurse from hell, I felt an uncontrollable need to push.

"Get this baby out!" I yelled.

"Pant, honey," the whey-faced nurse with ferret-like eyes urged.

"*You* pant." I countered.

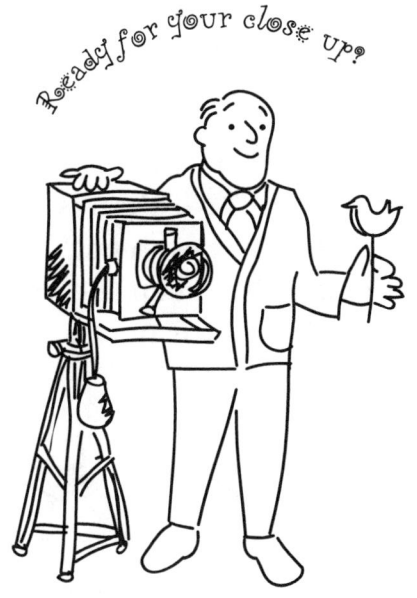

"We don't have to be unpleasant," she chided.

"*We* don't have to be anything," I growled between gritted teeth.

For twelve hours this creature had been telling me to do things. Now she had the gall to tell me *not* to push? She snagged a doctor unfortunate enough to stroll past the door.

"But I'm not an obstetrician," he whined. "I'm a PROCTOLOGIST!"

With my last ounce of strength, I grabbed him by his green scrubs. " I don't care if you do *nose* jobs," I said in a hoarse voice. "I want this baby out of me and I want it out NOW!"

He stuck his head between my legs and held out his hands just in time to catch a nine-pound squalling scrap of humanity.

Record one of the most body-stretching experiences in my life? No thanks. I've got all the reality I can handle. And even *without* recording his birth, we've managed to keep the tape rolling. That nine-pound bundle of joy is now a teenager!

Jane McBride Choate

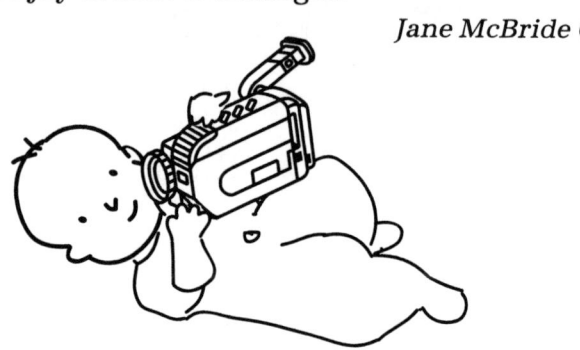

Don't Cry for Me Argentina!

A cold wind was whistling to proclaim the advent of winter in a suburb of Buenos Aires, Argentina, my husband's birthplace and my home since our marriage three years before. It was June 17, 1943, the equivalent of mid-December in the northern hemisphere.

I was expecting, and I knew it was time to go to the hospital. I called my husband at his office. "Oh Senora, el Senor Harry is out of the office at a business meeting," I was told. Oh well, many of my friends had declared their willingness to take me to the hospital when the time came. I made several calls, but that particular afternoon, I couldn't find even one of my volunteer friends at home.

I lumbered about, putting last-minute things in my bag, pondering what certainly seemed to be incipient birth pains. There was no reason I couldn't drive myself. More than a little piqued to have no one to share my adventure, I left word for Harry that I was on my way to the hospital.

Over the bumpy cobblestone street, in itself rough enough to bring on labor, I drove. Once on the Avenida, the main road to the city, I could plainly see the fresh bullet holes in buildings from the revolution that had just taken place. Revolutions occurred frequently enough to make us accept them rather casually, but I shuddered and hoped I wouldn't run into a military roadblock.

What I ran into instead as I drew near the Little Company of Mary Clinic (the "in" place for Americans to have their babies) was a would-be lothario in a convertible who was determined to play. On the wide and traffic-free boulevard he drove alongside my car and gestured to show me that he was smitten. When I sped up, he gave chase. When I lagged, he slowed as well.

This was a common game with young, romantic

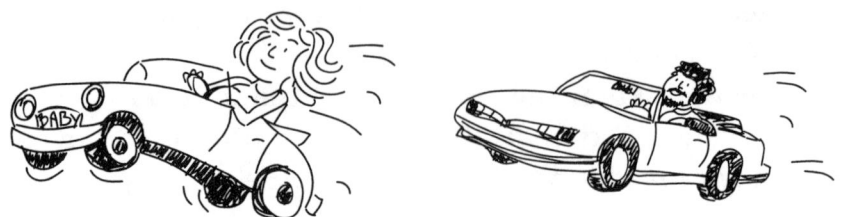

Argentines, and if the pursued showed indifference, the pursuer usually gave up and drove on. The thought of his reaction if he could see the rest of me, however, caused me to do the unthinkable. I laughed out loud. Of course, he mistook my amusement as agreement to meet him off the road.

About this time I arrived at the fin-de-siecle mansion, which housed the clinic. I slowed and pulled over to the curb at the entrance, lothario in hot pursuit. With the effort of extricating my bulk from the automobile, I missed my admirer's reaction to the drama unfolding before him: An expectant mother, greeted by a frenzied husband (who had received word from his office and hurried ahead), with a nurse and wheelchair in tow. It must have been a rather anticlimactic ending to his anticipated conquest. Mama Mia!

P.S. The blustery winds of June 17 were forgotten in the rosy dawn of the next day, when Harry and I were delighted to find that we had broken the Smith family thirty-year jinx of begetting only male children.

Patricia Ann Smith

A Far-Flung Story

I took childbirth classes with both my pregnancies and had read everything I could get my hands on. So during my second pregnancy, I felt that I was an educated mother and ready for anything!

I was about five days past my due date and starting to get a little anxious. I was resting on the couch when I felt a strange sensation between by legs! I thought my water had broken. I went to the bathroom to investigate. I pulled down my shorts and felt something tickling me. What in the...?

I reached down and encountered something slimy. I screamed! I snatched my hand away and as I did, I accidentally flung the slime onto the ceiling. It stuck! With my heart beating with fear, I looked at it for a minute and realized I had just lost my mucous plug and would soon be going into labor. I began to laugh so hysterically, I was crying.

My husband came in to make sure I was OK. I pointed to the ceiling, tears streaming down my cheeks, but for some reason my husband could not find the humor in a slimy blob stuck precipitously to the ceiling above his head.

In fact, my daughter is now nearly four-years-old, and this is the first time I'm sharing this story — I've finally pulled the plug on my most embarrassing moment.

Inga

To The Rescue

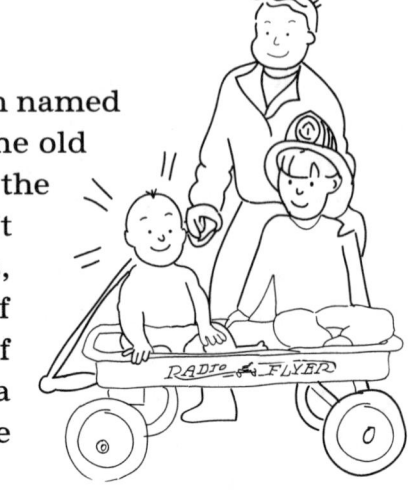

Our first child, a son named Jeff, was born back in the old days — 1966. Those were the days when women left their jobs at six months, not at six centimeters. Jeff was nearly four-and-a-half when our second child, a daughter, Ann, came along.

Having been "farm raised" in that generation, I don't remember telling Jeff that the baby was in Mommy's tummy. I remember talking to him about getting a new baby, that we'd get the cutest baby they had, and that it might even look like him! Further, I warned him that it might even be a girl!

"Labor Day" came. I had complained all day that my back hurt and I didn't feel well. A call to the doctor that evening confirmed everything. Jeff's daddy took him aside and told him it was time for Mommy and Daddy to go get the new baby. But Jeff, being sympathetic to Mommy, exclaimed in protest, "Oh, no, Daddy. Mommy doesn't feel good. Let her stay here and rest, and me and you go get the new baby!"

Betty Anslinger

Let Me Out

When my four children were very young, they took great delight in hearing about the events of their births. Some of my most precious memories are of those special quiet times when they would always make the request, "Tell me about when I was born."

My youngest son was ten days overdue when my membranes ruptured at home. When he was old enough to talk and understand, almost daily he would ask, "Mommy, tell me about the time when I was in your tummy and my big toe nail snagged a hole so I could get out!"

He would just beam with joy as I once again related the circumstances of this most special event.

Edie McAllister

Bottoms Up

Back when my father was a medical student, it was necessary for him to fly out of state to take his specialty boards. The problem was that he was scheduled to go only one day after my mother was due to give birth to me. She was afraid that she might go past her due date and that her husband would miss the birth of his first child.

Very much wanting to be present for the great event, my father was eager to speed things along. He telephoned the pharmacy and ordered a bottle of castor oil. It was an old-time remedy, not in the medical books, but worth a try. A short while later the doorbell rang. There, on the front step, was a bottle of castor oil with a note attached by a pink and blue ribbon. It read: "Bottoms up! With our compliments, your pharmacists."

My parents put the bottle aside and waited for nature to take its course, but still I made no move to enter the world. On the day before my father was to leave, my mother bravely swallowed several tablespoons of the gruesome liquid. It seemed only to make her feel queasy. She lay down to watch television, and my father headed off to continue studying for his medical boards. He had barely picked up a book, however, when things started to happen – fast. Less than two hours later, I was born.

Guess I was just what the doctor ordered!

Marianne Shine

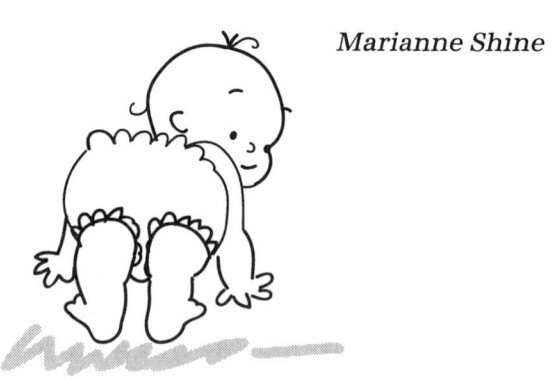

Table For Three

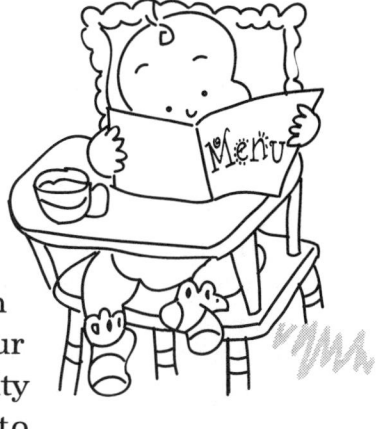

Several years ago, before our much-loved son came into our lives, my husband and I were at a crossroads. We had been trying to conceive for nearly seven years. Having exhausted all our options in the area of infertility treatment, we decided to contact an adoption agency and place our names on a waiting list to adopt a child. The agency warned that, because of the large number of couples on its list, we probably wouldn't hear anything for two or three years — maybe even four. We settled in for another long wait and tried to concentrate on other areas of our lives.

One glorious day within the first year, the phone rang. The agency was moving us, along with a few other couples, to the top of the list because we met some specific requirements of a certain birth mother who was due in six months. They asked us to prepare our biography right away and submit it. A few days later, the agency called back and said the birth mother had chosen us, based on our biography. We were elated. They had another bit of news, too — she was actually due in six *weeks*, not six *months*. A bit of a mix-up.

We were ecstatic, but we didn't want to get our

hopes all the way up. We'd heard so many stories of birth parents changing their minds at the last moment. We knew we should get busy preparing our home for a baby, but we'd been on such an emotional rollercoaster for so many years that we were afraid to believe that our dream really could come true. What if we dashed around, created a perfect nursery and got everything just right...and it didn't happen?

Another phone call from the agency, however, shifted me into baby mode fast. It seems there had been another small miscalculation: the baby was due in only *three* weeks. Now the pressure was on. We didn't own one stick of baby furniture and didn't have so much as a diaper. My head was swimming with thoughts of all the items that were necessary for proper care of a baby. I furiously made lists — baby bed, changing table, clothes, monitor, stroller, thermometer, rocker, diaper cream, booties, nail clippers. I was a whirling dervish. What if the baby came even earlier than the agency had predicted? Lots of mothers delivered two or three weeks early, didn't they? Yikes!

That night, my husband and I had dinner in a small, crowded restaurant. As we were discussing preparations for the baby, I became agitated with my spouse. He wanted to hold off on the shopping, saying we could do it later, maybe in a week or two. I knew what was going on. He still had all his defense mechanisms in place, and he just couldn't move ahead because it would be too devastating if the adoption fell through.

I, however, had passed that point with the last phone call. I was on a mission. My baby wasn't going to sleep in a cardboard box and have diaper changes on the floor. My baby was going to come home to organization and comfort. We had waited for too long, and I wanted everything to be just right. I had to make him see that time was of the essence. I had to make him feel the urgency I felt. I was near tears as I leaned across the table.

"Look," I blurted out in anger and frustration, *"we could have this baby any moment now!"*

As soon as my too-loud words were out, they seemed to just hang in the air. A sudden silence descended upon the nearby tables, and heads swiveled in our direction. I felt several pairs of eyes turn toward us and then travel down to my flat tummy. My husband and I sat like stone, with our eyes locked and our faces hot with embarrassment. As the other diners gradually went back to their own conversations, self-conscious giggling overtook us.

I can't imagine what the people seated near us were thinking, but I certainly didn't hear anyone tell the server, "I'll have what *she's* having!"

Paula Janicke

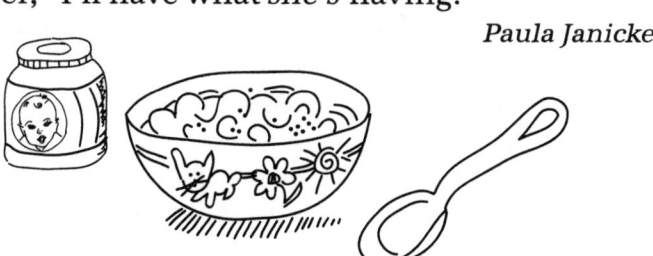

The Good Landlord

Back in 1949, my parents owned and lived in a large tenement building in the city. They were determined to keep things running smoothly... and to keep the tenants, whose rent money paid their steep mortgage, happy.

That first year was more difficult than my parents had anticipated. Night after night, their sleep was interrupted by some tenant who had a plumbing emergency, heating problem or malfunctioning major appliance. Still, no matter how late it was, my father, eager to please, would get out of bed and immediately take care of the problem.

The last week of October my mother was seven months pregnant with her first child. Something in the old building seemed to break or fall apart every other night. It was 2 a.m. on Halloween when Dad, exhausted from repairing a burst pipe on the third floor, finally climbed into bed and fell into a deep, deep sleep the moment his head hit the pillow.

An hour later, my mother was awakened by severe abdominal cramps. Because the baby wasn't due for two more months, she didn't suspect she was in labor...until her water broke.

Panicking, she shook my father and frantically whispered, "Lou, wake up! My water just broke!"

There was no response.

"Lou! Lou!" she repeated more loudly. "My water broke!"

Still no response.

"LOU!" She finally shouted, her voice rising several octaves. "MY WATER BROKE!"

My father slowly opened his eyes, sat up and shook his head to clear it. Calmly, he stood and walked out to the kitchen, as my puzzled mother watched. When he returned, he was carrying a huge pipe wrench.

"Whose water did you say was broken?" he muttered, his eyes still half-closed. "Is it that darned third floor again?"

My mother swears she laughed all the way to the hospital.

Sally Breslin

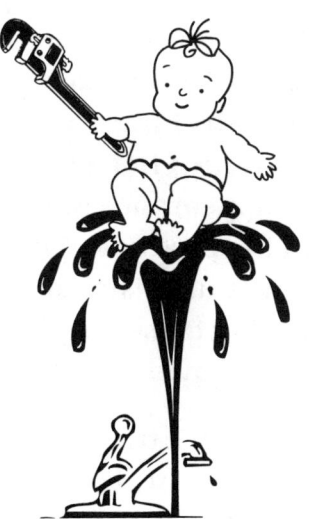

And The Award Goes To...

Plan A was to scream "Happy New Year!" while watching one of the many depressing blockbuster movies now showing.

But fate intervened with Plan B when my friend Diana starred in a private screening of "She's Having a Baby, Part II." Early in the morning on New Year's Eve, I was privileged to be part of the crew for this production, which had been some nine months in the making.

Driving in darkness toward the hospital, I remembered my original role five-and-one-half years ago during the birth of Diana's daughter. We walked the halls for miles, then sat in her delivery room as she slept fitfully between contractions. We coaxed that first baby into the world inch by inch, pleading and wheedling and cajoling her all the way. From the squished-to-death appearance of my left hand, I'd say my primary job in the production was that of Key Grip. Diana's husband was unmistakable as Best Boy. (I've always wondered what these people do as I watch their titles roll by on the movie credits, and now I know.)

Being part of that little drama was the most rewarding experience of my life, so I'd eagerly awaited the sequel. But when I arrived on the set, it was obvious that we were working from a different script this time around. My first clue was when I could hear Diana hollering all the way down the hall when I stepped off the elevator. In print, I can't get specific about what, exactly, she was hollering, but let's just say it wasn't "Happy New Year!"

Action was already under way. We'd bypassed the hall-walking, the chatting, the hand-squeezing, the contraction timing and were in the midst of full-scale labor. There were more tubes than I remembered from before, and more people in the room wearing concerned expressions. The baby had had a bowel movement, which could mean he was under stress, the doctor explained.

About this time the temperature suddenly seemed very warm. Numbers on the monitor indicating the strength of Diana's contractions began to glow orange. And how could my friend pant so readily, I wondered, when all the air had been sucked out of the room?

"I think I am going to faint," I announced, and was quickly steered out into the hall. Sheet white and soaked with sweat, I plopped into a wheelchair near the door. Some kind person—whom I can identify only by her shoes—brought me a wet cloth and a vomit dish before filling my request for the staff of life, a diet cola.

Hmmmm, what's wrong with this picture? My dearest friend was writhing in the next room, bravely trying to shove an eight-pound sack of wet cement through her loins, and I was the one who was feeling faint. She relied on me for emotional support, I responded by collapsing in a heap in the hallway, where I sucked down free soda through a hospital straw. There went my nomination for Best Supporting Actress.

Marching back in, I learned that further complications had been discovered. The baby's heart rate became unsteady. Within minutes, the doctor and Diana agreed that an emergency Cesarean section was called for. The room was emptied in a flash, leaving the baby's father and me standing there helplessly. He shook as he hugged me, "Everything will be OK," we said at the same time, whispering it like a prayer.

A mere seven minutes later, we greeted a seven-pound, fifteen-ounce, perfectly pink baby boy. I'd been on the scene all of an hour and ten minutes—boy, those sequels can wrap up fast! So on Dec. 31, I was truly blessed. Instead of watching a disaster on screen, I held a miracle in my arms.

What a perfect way to ring in the new year.

Marli Murphy
The Kansas City Star, 1998

Hands Up!

In February 1954 I was expecting our second child and because my husband was in the military, I was scheduled to give birth at the military hospital.

Even though my husband was away from home on military training maneuvers, I felt safe because he was to return before my due date. However, as all military wives know, every time your husband leaves home, the washer spins its last cycle, the kids get the flu and the car breaks down. So of course my water broke two weeks early and labor pains began. We had only lived in our duplex two months and had not become well acquainted with the people on the other side of us, but they were also military people. So the first thing I did was deposit our two-year-old son with the startled wife and I drove myself to the base.

As I was driving up to the gate I heard sirens and watched the gate close in front of me. A young corporal came out to meet me and advised that I could not enter because they were having a practice alert. I tried to explain my circumstances but he was in no way going to break orders.

The only thing I could do was to step out of the car. As I did, he raised and pointed his rifle at me and advised me to return to my car and leave. But then he saw my full figure, and he finally was convinced that maybe I *was* telling the truth. Knowing that he was not experienced in assisting with childbirth, he radioed ahead to some higher authority and I was allowed to go inside, with military escort. I went on to the hospital where I gave birth to our second son.

I found out later that the young corporal had radioed ahead to the hospital to tell them to expect me. His second point of action was to telephone his wife and tell her he had come near to helping deliver a baby.

In conclusion, mother and baby got through the experience just fine. Daddy caught a special flight home the next day, and number-one son had a wonderful time playing and sleeping over with the neighbor kids.

As the old mail saying goes, "Through rain or snow, through sleet or hail,..."

How about a new saying for laboring military wives? "Through sirens, through alerts, through pointed rifles . . . a woman in labor shall prevail!"

Wilma Bundridge

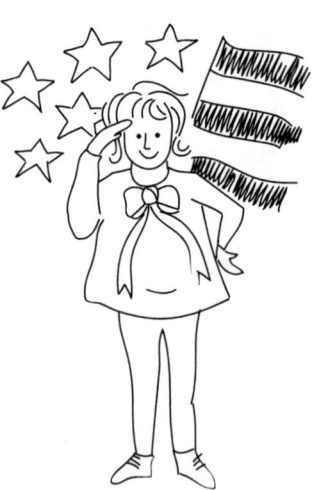

Chapter 3

Hospital Hilarity

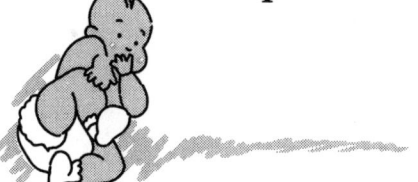

In The Dog House!

My wife was an aide on the maternity ward at the hospital. Late one night she heard sobbing coming from a new mother's room. She went in, and asked, "What's the matter, dear?"

"It's a boy," the new mother replied. "And I have four more at home. Even the darned dog is a male."

Frank James

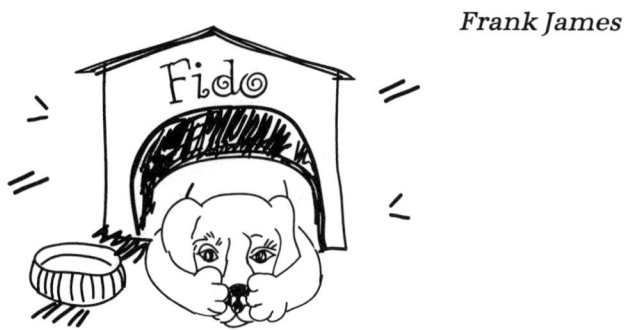

Nice Size Too

It was time to take my new son back to the hospital nursery. Though I would never tire of marveling at his fluttering fingers and crinkling face, I was wise enough to pace myself and take it a bit easy. This is the wisdom that comes after the fourth Cesarean.

Another new mother joined me near the nursery door. "Such nice dark hair!" she said. "Good size, too. How big was he?" she asked companionably.

"Eight pounds, six ounces," I answered. Then I slipped into the nursery to drop off Samuel. A moment later, I came out with another bassinet.

"Here's Peter," I said. "*He* was nine pounds, nine and a half ounces."

Luckily, my new acquaintance was near a chair.

Mary Beth Eckels

Baby Lotion

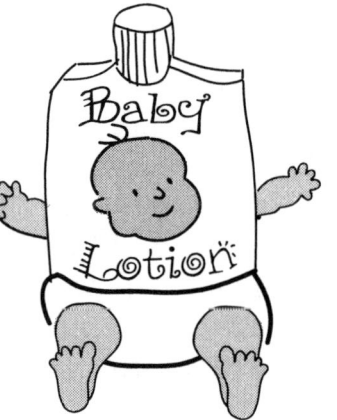

My son was born almost three weeks before his due date. He weighed a healthy seven pounds, but had no eyelashes or eyebrows. As is common with premature babies, he was covered with a thick white substance called vernix caseosa – a protective layer that shields the baby's skin from the amniotic fluid.

The nurses took him across the room to clean him up and perform the usual tests. I noticed that other nurses were joining them and, soon, several were crowded around the baby.

I began to be concerned. I summoned one of the nurses and asked whether the baby was all right. She assured me that he was fine and went on to explain that vernix caseosa is a wonderful natural emollient. It seems that the nurses were flocking from everywhere to "borrow" the much-sought-after skin cream from my baby to use on their hands and arms.

Now, that's baby lotion!

Vicki Miller

Some Other Guy

My father was a new preacher and was pacing with the other dads-in-waiting while my mother was in the delivery room of our hospital. He was told by the doctor that he was going to have a "big boy" because my mother had gotten so large. Ultrasound was not available in those days and the father of the baby was not allowed in the delivery room.

My father was about to receive the surprise of a lifetime.

A nurse emerged from the delivery room door. All eyes turned to him. Which father was the recipient of a bundle of joy?

"Mr. Perdew, you are the proud father of *two* little baby girls!"

My father responded with, "No, you must have me confused with someone else. I'm supposed to have *one big boy!*"

Lori Jane Perdew

Shock in the Waiting Room

I arrived late for the birth of my adopted daughter. I was told at the hospital that my husband was already in the delivery room and that I would have to stay in the waiting room while the baby was born. I went to the waiting room with the prospective fathers and felt a wee bit conspicuous. I was disappointed because it was I who should be in the delivery room. I wanted to see my child born, but traffic had delayed me. Thank goodness my husband worked only a few miles from the hospital and had gotten there in time.

The seven waiting men paced incessantly and opened and closed their magazines. I could identify with their nervousness. My husband and I were adopting our second baby, and our doctor had arranged permission for us to attend the birthing. Now here I sat, plenty upset and frustrated.

The doctor entered the room and smiled at me. "You have a beautiful eight-pound girl, and father and daughter are doing fine."

Pacing stopped and magazines closed as seven men stared at the doctor and me. My doctor saw the shock on their faces and quipped, "Medicine has advanced a long way, heh fellows?" Then he took my arm and walked me toward the recovery room. He snickered, "That ought to give them plenty to think about while they wait."

Florence B. Smith

In Stitches

It was late in the autumn season. A chill was in the air. But things were definitely warming up at home. I was a few days past my due date with my second child and felt those long-awaited contractions finally take over my body.

With "century" describing the length of my first labor, we casually arrived at the hospital expecting to have plenty of time for our second birth.

No sooner did we settle into the birthing room, unpack and flip the television on, than my contractions began intensifying. Everything was happening so fast!

The doctor, nurse, and other personnel came rushing in and our little daughter was quickly welcomed into this world.

Minutes later, during that tedious task of episiotomy repair, I noticed that everyone else in the room (except the doctor and me) was momentarily distracted by the television, which was above the doctor's head. I, too, glanced up to see what was so interesting. By this time, the doctor had realized

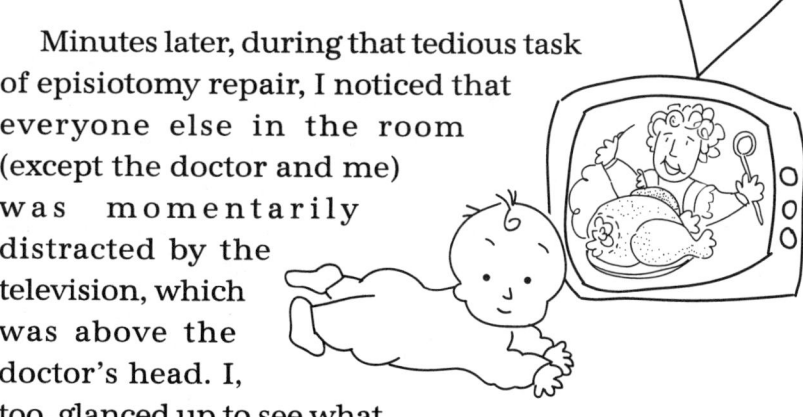

that our attention was on the television show, and she curiously glanced up over her shoulder. There, live and in person, was the famous Julia Child, mimicking the doctor. Only *her* sewing prize was named Tom...Tom turkey, that is. Julia was chatting away as she was stitching up ol' Tom in preparation for the Thanksgiving festivities.

Simultaneously, we all burst out in laughter, as Julia and her Thanksgiving turkey crashed *our* "stitching" party.

Cathi Freund

William Comes Home

My third son, William, was born in 1989. The hospital he arrived at was offering a free infant car seat at that time. The evening before he was due to leave, a nurse came in to tell me the car seat supply was running low and there might not be one available for him. I asked my husband to contact some friends to borrow one, since the hospital promised one when new supplies arrived. Everyone Ed contacted was unable to help him. He cheerfully informed me the next morning that he did not have a car seat, but not to worry — he had brought the baby bathtub.

Luckily the nurse arrived with the good news that

a car seat was ready for us. When we arrived home and had settled in, I asked him just how William was to have traveled home in the bathtub. His reply was that he had also brought along the duct tape.

I know men feel duct tape is necessary for survival, but I am glad in this instance, it was the second choice!

Rae Ann Kobylinski

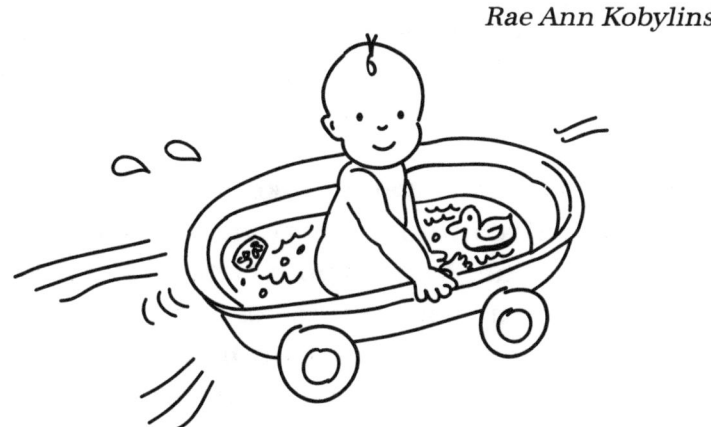

Baby Tooth

I began to suspect I was pregnant when my husband and I returned from Coney Island, where I'd satisfied an uncontrollable craving to eat a Kosher dill, which I promptly "got rid of" on the train ride home. The doctor confirmed my suspicions, stating that I was in my second month. He assured me that, when the time came, it would be an experience similar to having a tooth extracted.

Choosing a boy's name was easy. My husband and

maternal grandfather are Roberts. Robert would have been my name if I had been a boy. After some research, I decided that Lyle would be his middle name. Because Lyle means "from the island," the site of his conception, it was a definite fit.

My proposed due date was August 11. By August 25, with no baby in sight, I was as big as Buddha. My obstetrician promised that if I hadn't delivered by Labor Day, he would induce the birth. (Perhaps he meant to say "extract the tooth!")

On August 28, my water broke. By 8 p.m., with my contractions five minutes apart, my husband rushed me to the hospital. A dozen hours later, I was sweating it out in the labor room, my doctor had yet to make an appearance and the nurses' shift had changed. By 11 a.m., I was slaphappy on drugs and threatening to go home.

The nurse determined that the unborn baby had slung an arm over his head to impede his passage. Finally, she announced, "It's delivery-room time." Beneath the hot lights, I looked above the green mask hovering over me into the eyes of the doctor who'd compared this experience to a dental appointment! I gasped for breath as the room darkened.

Hours later, they brought me our son. The nurse pulled down his lower lip to reveal a unique development. Protruding from his gum was one long, jagged tooth!

Breast-feeding soon proved to be a struggle as I discovered my child was not so much a Robert as he was a Lyle, Lyle the Crocodile! However, my snaggle-toothed son was soon flourishing...from a bottle.

Rita Garitano

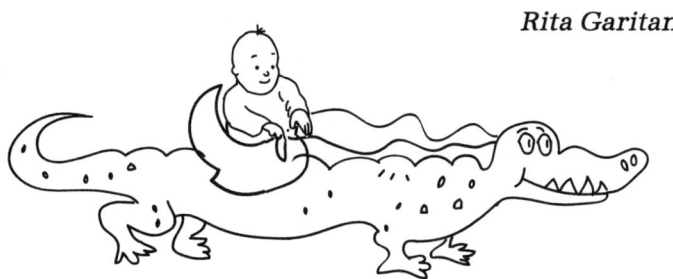

Half-Baked

Peering through the hospital nursery windows at a room full of newborns, four-year-old Ashley was anxiously looking for her brand-new twin brothers. As they were quite premature, we explained they were in a special place—warm and cozy in their incubators. She was very excited to bring them home until she spotted them.

"Dad, let's not take them home. Let's leave them here...they're not done yet!"

Pam Whitaker and Rawa Zari

Comedy Club

I followed the well-worn tread in the carpet around our dining room table trying to walk off the Braxton Hicks contractions, crying out at the onset of each one for my husband to keep time using his trusty stopwatch. We lumbered out to the car when the contractions were two minutes apart, even though my husband assured me, as he loaded the overnight bag into the trunk, that we were wasting our time. I was in false labor.

Friends who'd been sent home from the hospital with first children said labor can last for days; some went to dinner, some to the movies, some learned a foreign language before their children arrived. My husband, certain I was in false labor and would be sent home promptly, parked on the second floor of the hospital's garage, and left our overnight bag in the trunk.

"We won't need it," he said.

As he piloted me through the garage, I announced that I'd decided against having a baby. When the real labor started, I'd be an unworthy opponent.

"My wife *thinks* she's in labor," said my confident spouse as he ushered me into the hospital lobby where I sank my nails into the armrest of a plastic chair. The nurse who escorted us to an elevator asked if I would like a wheelchair, but my husband, who doesn't like to be any bother, dismissed her. "She needs to walk," he said. "Right, honey?"

No one was more surprised than I when the resident announced that I was dilated to five. "I need to keep walking," I said, perhaps thinking the condition would magically reverse itself. My husband stood mute, ghost-white, humbled.

Finally settled into my birthing room, the nurse inserted an IV needle into the vein on top of my right hand and plugged it with a little cork just as my doctor, a wanna be comedian, waltzed in wearing jeans, a polo shirt and latex gloves. "You're at six," he said, before jumping into a vaudeville act that included skits about a priest, minister and rabbi.

Between jokes I requested help delivering the baby, but Dr. Chuckles waved me off until my husband yelled, "I see the baby's head!" The doctor ran from the room to scrub up, and the nurse ordered me to stop pushing. My body, however, had its own agenda and it wasn't taking orders from anyone. The doctor rushed back into the room dressed in what looked like riot gear—a green suit, gloves and a face shield that ended up on the opposite side of the room after I lost control of my leg during a contraction.

Suddenly my outrageous doctor started waving his hands and clutching the air above me. While I was wondering what kind of new nonsense this was, all of a sudden he leaped up, grabbed my wrist and flung it to the bed. The cork from the IV tube had popped out, and blood was pulsating from my hand a la Monty Python.

It was during this confusion that the nurse inadvertently hit the television's "ON" switch, and soon everyone's attention turned from my daughter's reluctant entry into the world to the blare of the TV.

"Honey," I said to my husband, "I can't *do* this."

Dr. Chuckles turned from the television at my words, looked into my eyes and said, "Hey, I'm flattered...I know we are becoming close here, but no one's ever called *me* 'honey' during delivery before."

Finally, our baby girl made her grand entrance. My husband was panic-stricken when upon first perusal of our new bundle of joy he counted only nine toes. Calmly, the nurse assured me there were ten and asked what my husband did for a living.

"I'm an engineer," he said.

"Boy," said Dr. Chuckles, as he administered stitches, "I hope you didn't design *my* car." He then turned to me and said, "Hey, you get the no-belly prize."

Later, as my husband and daughter dozed on either side of me, I counted my blessings, *recounted my baby's toes and retrieved the missing IV cork from my tousled tresses. Oh yes, I also had time to regret not having my overnight bag — it was still safe in the trunk of the car.

Dorene O'Brien

Who Is That Masked Man?

Like any good husband I took the child birth classes with my wife; completed the class and received my certificate of completion. We awaited the big day. Just so happens the big day turned out to be THE BIG NIGHT. At 2 a.m. my wife woke me. I grabbed the suitcase, got my wife, secured my certificate from the birth class and went to the hospital. I was ready.

Upon arrival I was instructed to put on a mask and gown before entering the delivery room. After I got dressed I confidently entered the room. I began to take charge as I started to question the physician working with my wife.

He looked me square in the eye and asked "First child?"

He proceeded to explain (while laughing) that the mask I was wearing was supposed to be placed horizontally across my mouth and nose, while I had placed the mask vertically, covering my whole face.

Needless to say, my confidence was shot and from that point forward the doctor was in complete control.

Richard E. Wallace, Jr.

In The Swim

Competitive swimming was the focus of my family's activities, involving my sisters, brother and me for most of our growing-up years. Even as an adult, I stayed involved with the sport, coaching a local swimming team during the summer of my pregnancy with my parents' first grandchild.

When my daughter arrived, my family visited my hospital room bearing gifts: a tiny girls' swimming suit with matching terrycloth robe, an infant-sized "beach" towel emblazoned with the Olympic rings, and a huge plastic wading pool, which by all accounts was difficult to manage in the crowded elevator.

The gifts may have foretold my daughter's future. She attended Indiana University on an athletic scholarship–from the women's varsity swimming team.

Mary-Lane Kamberg

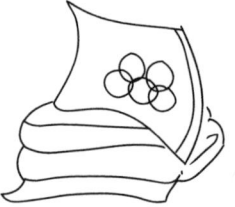

Double Whammy

In that fateful year of 1950, I felt as though I had a football team in my stomach. I had prepared things for only one baby. But two minutes after my baby was born, a second baby emerged. My husband remembers in my shocked state, I said, "Now what in the world am I going to do with *this* one?"

Irene E. Norwood

Pins and Needles

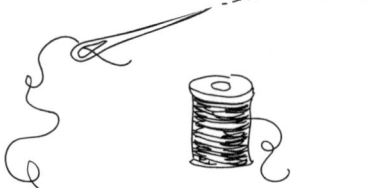

After three false alarms, labor had finally started. My husband and I were anxiously awaiting the birth of our second child. But, after fourteen hours of labor, the doctor had to perform an emergency C-section. We were on pins and needles. Was the baby okay?

With great aplomb, the doctors started the C-section, and before I knew it, the doctor lifted the baby up and brought it over for me to kiss quickly on the forehead before whisking it away.

My husband yelled over to the attending pediatrician, "What is it?"

"It's okay." He answered as he examined the baby.

"NO, what *is* it?" My husband inquired again.

"It's just FINE," the pediatrician repeated with his voice a little louder.

Finally, the nurse intervened. "No, doctor," she said, "They want to know what *sex* it is."

"Oh... ," said the doctor, "it's a girl!"

Wendy Lee Klenetsky

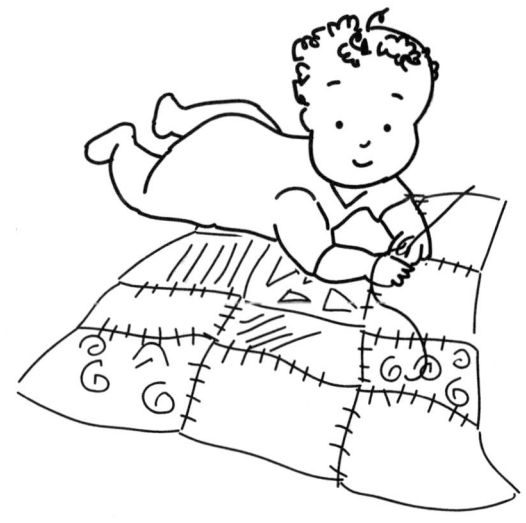

Chapter 4

Baby Banter

Got Milk?

With my third child, I decided to breast-feed. I hadn't been successful at breast-feeding my first two children, but I was determined to go through with it this time. I quit my job so that I wouldn't have to worry about nursing as a working mother.

At the hospital, I had been told that my ten pound son probably would require a feeding every three to four hours. I thought I must have been misinformed, however, because he was nursing every two hours. I didn't realize that breast-fed babies eat more frequently.

With a newborn, a two-year-old and a three-year-old, there was never a dull moment. One day, when the baby began to cry, my younger daughter took up his cause. She informed me that the baby wanted some milk and that I should bring those "things" so he could eat.

My older daughter, too, chipped in with her 2¢ worth, "Mom, bring them bottles – NOW!!"

Alesia J. Robinson

Look, Don't Touch

My daughter recently became a first-time mother. When her baby was three-weeks-old, my daughter called me at work to report that she had taken her baby girl with her to the grocery store. It seems that she had gotten more than she'd bargained for.

"Mom, all these ladies came over to look at her! Then they wanted to touch her. They tried to touch her hands, and then they tried to touch her face. I don't care if they look, but I didn't want them to touch, so I decided to say, 'Oh, please don't touch her...she's brand new!'"

Kathy Hinson

Cowa"bungie"!

It took an hour to prepare my first child for his first stroller outing.

Into the diaper bag went proof of my new-mother diligence: diapers, powder, undershirt, outfit, booties, blanket, bottle of formula, bottle of water, pacifier, rattle, teething ring. (In case my two month old started to teethe in the next twenty minutes.)

Then I began to prepare him. Diaper, undershirt, little blue pants, little blue shirt, little blue booties, blue receiving blanket, in which I bundled him before placing him in a heavier blanket. It was blue.

Almost out the door, I realized I had forgotten his bonnet. Earaches! Back we went, emerging only after the little blue ear-flapped hat had been secured beneath his tiny chin.

After releasing the seat lever so he could lay flat, I laid him down beneath the awning. I couldn't see him in there once I began to push, so I stopped to check on him in the middle of the first block, saw he was asleep, and began to relax.

When we reached our first corner, I tilted the stroller back, easing it down the curb as my eyes scanned for cars. Doubling my pace to get us quickly across, I pushed the stroller up the opposite curb and proceeded walking into the next block.

That's when I heard someone cry, "The baby!"

What baby? What errant mother wasn't keeping an eye on her child? I looked around but saw no toddler toddling into the road. What baby?

I was stopped anyway, so I rounded the stroller to check on my own son. I peeked inside. He wasn't there.

Frantically, I looked back across the intersection. And there, lying in the gutter, were the blankets, the booties, the bonnet and...the baby.

Apparently when I tilted the stroller onto its rear wheels to get down that first curb, I was simultaneously checking the traffic. He was taking that opportunity to silently slide, head first, into the street.

Oh, he was fine. But it seems I had packed every single thing he might possibly need for this carefully planned outing except one: a little blue bungee cord.

Terri Watrous Berry

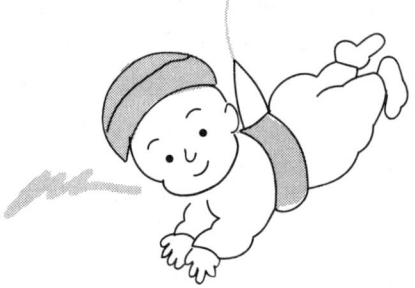

Boomerang Children

We baby boomer mothers may just have created a generation of baby wombers. Here's how: Our children grow up and go off to college (preferably prestigious ones), graduate, and just as we parents are beginning to enjoy being a couple again, the kids return. Yup. They boomerang back! After all, what's not to like here?

Now that I think back, I should have recognized the prenatal signs. First, it took almost three years to conceive our oldest. Even then, she didn't want to leave the safety of her being no more than a glimmer in our eyes and heart. Then, during my pregnancy, in her embryonic ecstasy, she most likely approved of my style sense and, right then and there, decided she would grow only slightly taller than I so she could also borrow my clothes.

Another sign appeared by her being three weeks late. And why not? She was comfortable. Nice room. Good, healthy meals and no household responsibility. All right, maybe space was a little tight, especially during the last trimester — but compared to a New York City studio, not all that bad! Besides, there was no one yelling at her yet to neaten things up. Best of all, there was no monthly rent to come up with and no security deposit required. Yes, those gestation days were the good 'ole days she just didn't want to give up.

Had I only interpreted other signals as well: on Monday mornings she was never "ready" to go back to school; she hated camp; and she always preferred that her friends come to our house to play.

Ah, here's the rub. Maybe we moms do too good a job creating a secure, warm, everything-at-your-fingertips environment for our children.

In comparison, is the outside world really that unsafe...frightening...expensive? And even if it is, how can we be angry with our kids for learning one of life's most important lessons: There's no place like home.

Wilma Davidson

Blame it on the Baby

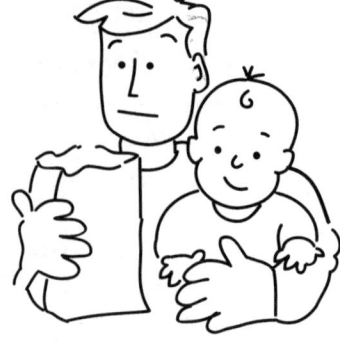

When my son was a couple of weeks old, he and I went to Wal-Mart to pick up a prescription for his mother. As we were waiting in line with several other people, my son, as babies will do, rather noisily released some gas.

A lady, somewhat hard of hearing, who I would guess to be well over eighty years of age, walked toward me and smiled. She grabbed my arm and said loudly, "THAT'S OKAY, SON, JUST BLAME IT ON THE BABY!" Of course, all of the rest of the people in line started laughing at the red-faced new father and his 'noisy' little baby.

Michael Barnes

Enough is Enough!

I didn't know I was carrying twins until they were born, two months before the due date in 1971. Now, two babies instead of one was a big surprise for my husband, Bill, and me. But it was an exceptionally new and difficult-to-understand concept for our almost two-year-old son, Paul.

I came home from the hospital with photographs and stories of the new brothers and an estimated two weeks to prepare our family for a new and different lifestyle. While we waited for the brothers to grow big enough to come home, the concept of two came up frequently in our mother-child conversations — two cookies, two balls, two teddy bears, two trips down the slide. I was beginning to think this wouldn't be so difficult.

Three weeks passed and the hospital staff informed us that we could bring Nicholas home. It was a big day. Nanny and Aunt Kate arrived to watch Paul. Bill and I got dressed up to go to the hospital. We returned with the first brother, Nicholas. It was a busy time, and we were delighted that Paul seemed to be adjusting to our growing family.

Two weeks later the hospital informed us that we could bring Billy home. Once again, Nanny and Aunt Kate arrived. Bill and I got dressed up to go to the hospital. We returned and life took on a hectic pace, but Paul seemed to be taking it in stride.

Just a few weeks later, my mother decided that I needed a break. So Nanny and Kate volunteered to baby-sit all three children and give Bill and me a night on the town. By this time, I was ready for a night out. I spaced my preparations throughout the day, washing my hair, taking a bubble bath, doing my nails and setting our evening clothes on the bed.

I noticed that Paul was not in his usual shadow position. I went to look for him in every room of the house, knowing full well that there was no way he could have unlocked the doors. I backtracked to his bedroom, and a noise in his closet caught my attention. I opened the door and found him sitting on the closet floor, his eyes filled with tears.

"Honey, what's the matter?" I asked. "You know Nanny and Aunt Kate will be here any minute." His big green eyes looked into mine and he said, "Please, Mama, don't bring home any more babies."

Ellen Michna

All American

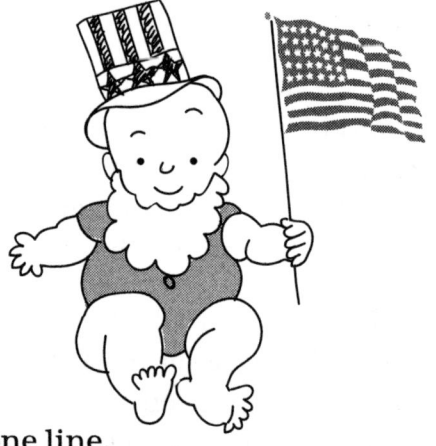

When I was nine or ten years old, my younger brother Ryan was born. One day shortly thereafter, I overheard my mother recanting the birth story to someone on the other end of the telephone line.

All I heard my mother say was, "Ryan was breech."

I yelled back, "No he's not, Mom! He's American!"

Tosha Sloan

Milky Way

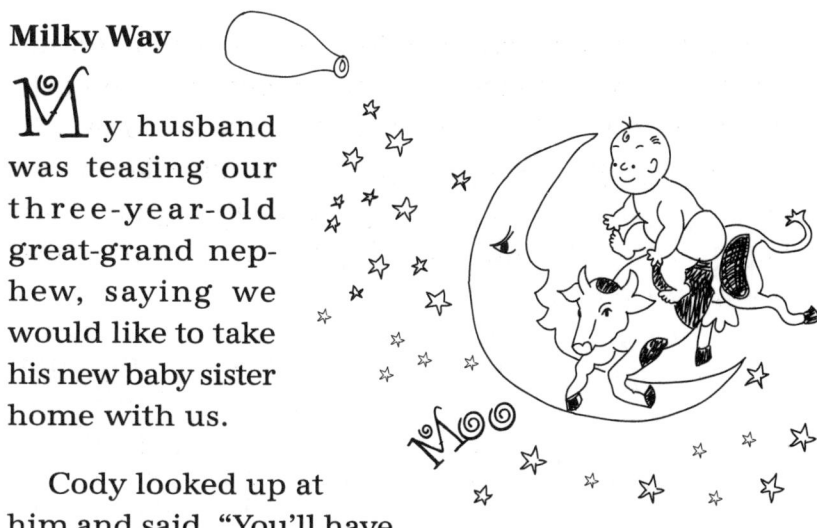

My husband was teasing our three-year-old great-grand nephew, saying we would like to take his new baby sister home with us.

Cody looked up at him and said, "You'll have to take Mommy, too, 'cause she has the milk!"

Irene E. Norwood

BYOB

There's a growing trend toward birth parties. These are not to be confused with birthday parties, which are a mother's annual reminder that she once endured indescribable discomfort. Birth parties, on the other hand, take place while a mother endures indescribable discomfort.

I watched such an event one day as mothers gave birth on "Oprah." These "coming out" parties featured cake and champagne, dancing and dining. In one instance a crowd of relatives cheered, "Push it out, push it out, wa-a-ay out!" I fully expected the woman to give birth to Brett Favre.

One mother-to-be even received a manicure. Hmmmm. Cuticles were the last thing on my mind when I was in the delivery room.

Unlike those birth mothers whose makeup and hair were flawless, I looked as indisposed as I felt. My labor began after I went to bed, and putting on my face before driving to the hospital was not an option. Consequently, pictures taken of me in my hospital bed are downright scary.

On her way out the door, a woman on the program reminded her husband, "Don't forget the cake!" As I recall, I had more of a craving for morphine.

When asked why she had a birth party, another woman said it was a way of celebrating life. It also gives guests a unique opportunity to observe you having one heck of a bad hair day.

But, surprisingly, everyone on the program seemed glad they had commemorated the occasion with a fiesta. Could there be something to this new fad? If I ever find myself in a birthing room again, maybe I should host an informal get-together, too. Wearing my trendy hospital gown, I wouldn't have to worry about being overdressed.

But what would we do for entertainment? I know—

charades! With teeth clenched and eyes bulging, I could easily mime the movie title, "Misery."

When my son was born, I was reluctant to let everyone hold my precious bundle. If I ever do throw a birth party, it would have to be a BYOB. Bring Your Own Baby.

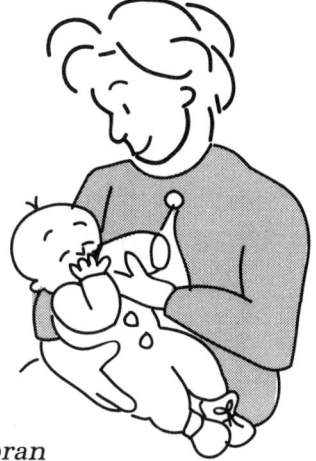

Lois Corcoran

Babies By The Schedule

If you run into any trouble, don't forget the Dr. Spock book. It's on top of the TV," my wife, Jackie, called to me, as a nurse guided her down the hall to maternity. I gave an indulgent smile and a confident wink.

We were going to have our fourth baby, and the one thing I was prepared against was trouble.

A week earlier, she had said, "Let's have Mom come up. She just loves to take care of the kids."

"Nonsense," I had said, "your mother lives in Florida now, and we live in Delaware. I'll simply take a week's vacation and handle it myself. I have a schedule. Cereal for breakfast, playtime till lunch, then soup and a sandwich, more playtime, visit you in the afternoon, come back home, give them dinner and a bath, put them to bed and read to them. It's that simple. I can do it alone, without assistance. Now that's that."

Now I was on my own. Just me and my schedule.

I left the hospital and got in the car. The three kids, in unison, all cried, "Where's Mommy?" Joe, a friend I had brought along to watch them, smiled.

"She's going to have the baby. I've already explained all of that to you."

"Can't we wait here while she has it?" asked Cecilia, the five-year-old. "No, we can't," I answered. Billy, the two-year-old cried, "Mommy, Mommy!"

At home, I gave them dinner, a bath, and read to them. Everything according to schedule. It was now 8 p.m. Should be hearing from the hospital anytime now.

Suddenly a piercing scream came from the bedroom. I dashed into the room, turned on the light, and saw Connie, the three-year-old, sitting up in bed. She had a querulous expression and seemed ready to emit another ear-shattering blast.

"What happened?"

"Cecilia touched me."

"Is that all? I thought you were being kidnapped. Now go to sleep."

After waiting until 5 a.m. and still not hearing from the hospital, I decided to sneak a cat nap. As I was pulling up the covers, the phone rang.

"A girl," the doctor said.

"Is everything...is..?"

"Everything is fine. Go back to bed."

"Back to...oh yes, thanks doctor." I hung up the phone and turned and saw six little eyes staring at me.

"Was that Mommy?" asked Cecilia.

"No, that was the doctor. Mommy just had a little girl. You have a new sister."

"But I wanted a boy baby," she said.

"So did I," said Connie.

"Puppy," said Billy.

An hour later (it took me that long to find Billy's clothes and dress him) and still sleepless, I opened the cereal box.

"Let's have pancakes," Connie said.

"Let's have eggs," Cecilia said.

"Pizza...pizza," cried Billy.

They settled for French toast.

After breakfast I put the dishes into the sink, the dirty clothes into the washer, and sat back to enjoy a second cup of coffee and the day-old Sunday paper. These small pleasures were interrupted by a low grinding noise coming from the washer, followed by a deluge of soapy water. I frantically turned the dial.

"Lift up the top and it will stop," Cecilia said. She was right.

"You put too many clothes in and too much soap," she added. As I started yanking out clothes, I heard her mutter something to her sister. It sounded like, "Gee, daddies can't do anything."

That afternoon I pulled into the hospital parking lot. "Wait here with Joe. I won't be long," I said to Cecilia.

"Why can't we come?" she asked.

"They don't allow kids."

"They don't allow kids?"

On my way to the maternity ward I practiced positive thinking.

"How's the schedule working?" Jackie inquired.

"Fine, but when are you coming home?"

"Wednesday. Two more days. Can you manage?"

" Have no fear, your husband's here," I said, not too positively. Shouts of "Mommy, Mommy" floated through the partly opened window. Looking out, we saw Joe and the three kids standing on the lawn about twelve feet below.

"I saw Daddy through the window," called Cecilia.

"Daddy wouldn't make pancakes, and he broke the washer," called Connie.

"Mommy, Mommy...puppy," cried Billy.

"How come they don't like kids?" yelled Cecilia.

Jackie smiled down and threw kisses as she brushed away a tear.

The next day, while Joe baby-sat, I headed for the supermarket. With the assistance of four clerks, the manager, and a fluttery middle-aged woman in a purple miniskirt, I purchased the week's groceries. Then I headed for the hospital, parked the car, took the hospital steps two at a time, and breezed down the hall to maternity.

"Well, my dear, what time should I pick you up tomorrow?"

"I should be ready at 10 a.m."

That night my schedule met with a few minor setbacks. I burned the TV dinners, the bath water ran over, Billy tore Connie's Cinderella book, and all three of them refused to go to sleep. They kept threatening "to tell Mommy."

The next morning I awoke before the children and had their clothes laid out and their breakfast waiting for them.

"Wait here with Joe while I pick up your mother and the baby," I said.

When we returned home, the kids argued about who was going to take care of the new baby. Although three wonderful kids had come to the premature realization that fathers are indeed fallible, the experience also brought out their tender and humane instincts. They were even willing to fib for me, their dear sweet ol' Dad. I distinctly heard Cecilia say, "Gee, Mommy, Daddy is really a good cook." Connie and Billy both agreed. A little too enthusiastically, I thought.

Although my schedule wasn't a complete disaster, from that day on, I was on the best of terms with my lookin'-better-by-the-minute mother-in-law.

William T. Ficka

But There's No Instruction Book

The young couple in the house across the street were thrilled when their first baby arrived. Still, like many first-timers, Mom and Dad thought they were all thumbs when handling their not-so-tiny daughter.

I did my best to help and reassure Melody that she was doing a great job, but one day I dropped by and found her in tears.

"I'm so tired all the time," she sobbed, "and Tyson is just no help at all!"

So to cheer her up, I wrote this for the reluctant father.

How to Change a Diaper.

1) Should the infant in your care be screaming 'fit to bust' for no apparent reason, sniff current diaper. One sniff should be enough.

2) Place child in safe place. The floor's good as he/she can't fall off. Assemble equipment:

a) Waterproof changing mat
b) Fresh diaper (or two — allow for accidents)
c) Wet wipes or cotton wool swabs and bowl of warm water

d) Cream for baby's - uh - rear end
e) Disposable bag to conceal the evidence

A waterproof apron for you is a good idea, but, much as you may feel the need for one, a gas mask is not. Do you want to traumatize the poor kid for life?

3) Place infant so it is lying on its back on the changing mat. Remove the baby's clothing and move it out of the way. Take a deep breath. Now unfasten the soggy diaper, holding onto the baby's feet as you do so. Whatever you do, don't let go of those feet. All babies have an overwhelming desire to splash their toes in the contents of their diaper. If they do manage to cover their feet and legs with it, you'll be amazed how far they can propel the stuff.

4) Holding onto the baby's feet, fold the filthy diaper in half so you can clean the affected areas. Grab a wet wipe or dampened cotton swab and wipe the whole area until all is clean and sweet. Do not leave the bowl of water within the little darling's reach. Babies may not be able to grab their own toes, but leave something messy or dangerous where they can get it, and you can guarantee they will.

5) Using cotton wool swab, dry carefully, paying plenty of attention to all the folds and creases. Just think — if you live long enough, one day someone will have to do this for you, so be gentle.

6) Lift the baby slightly by the feet so you can pull out the dirty diaper. Slightly, I said; you don't want to scare the poor child by standing it on it's head. Drop the diaper and the used cleaning materials into the disposal bag, which you have left standing open. You haven't? Well you'll have to work out how to open a plastic bag while holding a baby by the feet with one hand and a diaper full of something unmentionable in the other; I haven't the slightest idea how it's done.

7) Lay the baby back down on the changing mat while you unfold the clean diaper. The part with the pretty pictures should go across the kid's belly; the other end, with the sticky tabs, goes at the back. Babies really enjoy lying on the mat and kicking their legs around at this stage, and yours will probably grin and gurgle at you. Take this opportunity to smile and babble back, but don't lean too close. If you do, you may find you have to change your clothes. Even girl babies can squirt remarkable distances; as for the ones with the hose-pipe attachment....

8) Grab those waving feet again and gently elevate the rear end. Now slide the back of the clean diaper underneath and lay the baby on top of it. Still holding the feet, put some cream on your fingers and smooth

it on. No, not on the kid's face. Use your imagination.

9) At this point, some babies decide they need to relieve themselves again. Stand by with that extra diaper. If you're lucky and the kid in question doesn't, pull the front end of the diaper between it's legs, unstick the fastening tabs on the back end and stick the back end to the front. If the tabs appear to already be attached to the end that comes through the baby's legs, you've put the thing on backwards, and you obviously weren't listening at #7. Pay attention. The part with the tabs should be under the kid. You unfold them, bring them around the sides, and stick them to the part with the pictures, which should be across the kid's belly. Is that clear enough for you? Sheesh, anyone'd think you needed to be a rocket scientist to change a diaper....Oh, by the way, don't get the cream on the tabs or they'll never stick unless you use duct tape.

10) Finally! Dress the baby again and put it in a safe place, like the floor, crib or playpen. Now go and find a beer — you probably need one. I certainly do.

After we had shared a laugh over my instructions, I told Tyson the next installment is going under the title "Burping for Beginners." He just can't wait.

Lynn Jenks

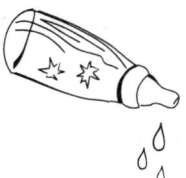

Lights, Camera, Action!

"Can we stop by tomorrow and shoot some film?" asked the talent agent. She was looking for a mother and baby "team" for a TV commercial, and someone had recommended us during our stay in Poland.

Of course, I was flattered, and not only vain enough to want to be on TV, but also greedy enough to fantasize about a modeling contract for my daughter. In fact, for the rest of the day, every time I caught a glimpse of Juliet's long curly eyelashes, I thought, "new car."

The next day, right on cue, Berta the talent agent swept into our living room. As the lights and cameras went up all over, the thrill of being "discovered" hung in the air.

"Can Juliet sit by herself?" asked Berta, while directing me to seat her on a blanket.

"Uh, we've been working on that...."

Meanwhile, Juliet's legs were locked like steel poles, and I couldn't coax her onto the floor. Finally, her legs gave out and she settled into a sitting position. Then she toppled over.

"Who's the commercial for?" I asked, trying to change the subject.

"Gerber," she said.

"We love Gerber! Juliet, don't you just adore their carrot soup?"

It was hard to be hopeful when the shoot was finished. Berta told me we were up against ninety other pairs. And Juliet just didn't have what it took - she definitely wasn't sitting by herself.

"If the agency is interested, you'll hear something today." By 5:00 p.m., I was sure we were has-beens.

Imagine my surprise when Berta called ten minutes later. After asking our dress sizes, she said, "We've narrowed it down to you and another party. A car will pick you up tomorrow morning at 11:00!"

That evening, I got the makeover of a lifetime. A team of beauticians worked with steely precision, coloring my hair coal-black, strapping me into a tanning bed and filing my nails into a French manicure.

Not that it mattered.

When we got to the studio the next day, I was met by a sultry, dark-haired model.

"Where's your baby?" I asked.

"Right there," she said, pointing at my daughter.

I'd been bumped, and who could blame them?

The professional model paraded in front of the agency's decision makers, holding Juliet in her arms and making kissy-poo faces at her with the kind of grace I never could have mustered. I would have tripped over the tripod.

Juliet cooed delightedly at her new mother. No separation anxiety today, I noticed — while I checked out the competition. There lay chubby baby Bart on the carpet, man handling a plastic donut. He just didn't seem—how shall I put this delicately? — very Gerberish. Who knew he'd crawl off with a modeling contract for a 30 second commercial on Polish television?

Juliet may not be the next Gerber baby, but she got paid $225.00 for three hours of work. That's enough for a new copy of Pat The Bunny, a snowsuit and a whole shelf of Gerber carrot soup.

Tara McKelvey

A "Case" of Mistaken Identity

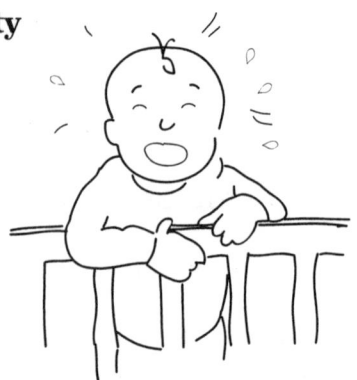

My newborn, colicky daughter, Kaylee, insisted my wife and I train all summer for the next ski season by doing deep knee bends. The toughest of coaches, Kaylee would scream if they were not of Olympic depth. When they were, she immediately quieted. But if we slacked off by trying to sneak in a half hearted dip, she would bellow again.

If we could hold out through the workout, Kaylee would eventually sleep. I'll never forget the peacefulness of her sleeping hours. Yet after weeks and months — which seemed months and years — there weren't enough sleeping hours to offset the screaming ones; we were exhausted. We had been worn down far enough that we were not above collapsing with our momentarily sleeping babe into our own bed, fearful that even a delicate placing into her crib would bring on the child's infernal howling.

Over time, as we grew used to being awakened in the night, we took turns changing diapers and, of course, deep knee bends. Yet even when her crying stopped, we knew, we had bought only an insignificant amount of peace and rest. One night when my wife and I were especially tuckered out we heard Kaylee crying, and I reluctantly conceded that it was my turn.

Let me repeat, we were especially wiped out.

I stood like an automaton and, mostly asleep, lifted what I thought was Kaylee's pudgy body from beside my wife in our bed, thinking we had earlier given in to the sin of master bedroom/infant encroachment. Immediately, beside our bed, I went to work perfecting my stem Christie in the sleepy fashion of Jean-Claude Killy. Down and up and down and up and down, in the pitch of an unasked hour. For a while all was quiet, like the peace of being the last skier of the day skimming down a deserted run.

Then I heard the crying!

There are defining moments in each life which make a man and a couple who they are; this was not one of those. You see — the crying was not coming from the 'master bedroom' — not from the pudgy child I believed with all my aching legs that I had calmed in my arms; rather, it emanated — from another room in the house.

The baby's room!?!

I looked closer at the sleeping child in my arms.

In my semi-conscious state, I had picked up a pillow. Embarrassed, yet smiling — like a skier who falls flat in front of the chalet — I lay down the pillow and reported to the coach to practice still more deep knee bends.

Bill Rudolph

Thank God for Chocolate Chip Cookies

When I first met my son-to-be, I saw a slim, scared-looking boy with flyaway brown hair and bright blue eyes. Holding himself stiffly straight, he thrust out his hand and said, all in one breath, "My name is Jimmy I'm seven-years-old and I've got big feet."

The caseworker brought him in and began explaining procedures for this initial visit. Jimmy sat quietly, looking around. Finally, his nose twitching, he burst out, "Chocolate chip cookies! I think I'm gonna like it here."

He did, and over the years he has brought me joy, heartache — and three grandchildren!

Doris Land Mueller

Waistline Woes

We were visiting relatives who had a four-year-old daughter, Lauren. She carried her favorite doll with her everywhere. Trying to make polite conversation, my husband said, "Lauren, how old is your baby?" Evidently, Lauren had overheard her mother talking to friends who were new mothers because she looked down at her waistline and replied, "Six months old...and I still haven't lost my stomach."

Connie Daarud

Missing Something?

After listening to the relatives admire and comment about her new baby brother, Ashley chimed to her mother, "Daddy still has his nose."

Perplexed at this sudden observation, the mother replied, "Yes, Ashley, but how did this come up?"

"Well..., Grandma said the baby sure had his Daddy's nose!"

Wynema Colson

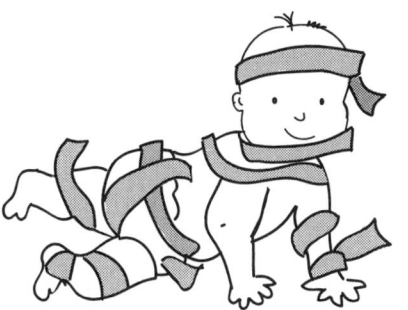

Resourceful

My dad was watching our five-month-old son at our house. It was time to change our baby's diaper, but Grandpa discovered there were no diapers in the house. Because baby's pants were especially soggy, the situation needed immediate attention.

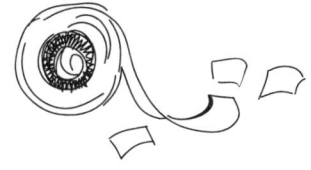

So what did this first time grandpa do? He cleaned up the baby and wrapped him in a good old receiving blanket. Then he realized he still needed something to hold the blanket in place. What to use? He ran out to the garage and grabbed the duct tape.

He wrapped his happy grandson in his new invention — The Receiving Blanket Diaper! Complete with never-fail duct-tape.

Rest assured, the blanket did not come loose all day.

S. Hayes

Express Delivery

They say swift births run in families. On the Danish side of my family, this certainly seems to be true.

My great aunt was lying in a hospital bed with the early signs of labor. She asked the nurse to help her get to the bathroom. Instead, the nurse brought her a bedpan. The result wasn't exactly the nature's offering my great aunt had been expecting. A moment later, my uncle appeared — in the bedpan, of course.

Another Danish aunt of mine felt her labor pains begin one afternoon while her husband was at work. Because it was during wartime, gasoline and cars were rationed to only a select few. She decided to ride her bike to the hospital, where her husband would meet her. By the time she arrived at the emergency room, however, her vehicle had turned into a bicycle built for two. She was standing on the bicycle pedals, and her baby's head was resting on the seat.

Marianne Shine

The Shape of Things to Come!

Soon after having my second child, I embarked upon an exercise program to lose the weight I had gained during pregnancy. In addition to lifting light weights, my exercise routine included a brisk walk every day. But, shedding the pounds was proving to be much harder than it had been after my first baby.

One day, accompanied by a visiting grandpa, I hoofed it downtown with the new baby in a stroller. We walked around, enjoying the beautiful spring weather and admiring the shop windows. In the window of one store, something caught my eye. Grandpa suggested that I go in and take a closer look while he waited outside with the baby. Grateful to get a break from exercise, I went in.

Immediately, a very smiley salesclerk was on my

heels, asking whether I needed assistance. I replied with the usual: "Just browsing." With that, he stepped closer and asked, "When's the big day?" I looked around and realized the clerk was referring to me — and my belly.

With a big smile, I answered, "At this rate, it could take months, maybe years." I'll never forget the look on his face.

Marianne Shine

Sympathetic Ear

As a new mother, when my infant son came down with a cold and fever, I called a health care hotline for advice.

The nurse on the other end of the line was very helpful, not to mention sympathetic to how my son was feeling.

She asked questions about his symptoms, all the while showing great concern.

She then asked what his temperature was. I told her 102 degrees.

"Poor little guy. How awful!" she responded. " And how are you taking it?"

I told her, "Not too good. I haven't gotten a good night's sleep in over three nights!"

There was a short silence before she blurted out, "No! No! I mean how are you taking your baby's temperature?"

Bonnie Jewell

Full of Flavor

One day as I was nursing my newborn, my three-year-old son was nearby. Looking thoughtful, he pointed to my chest and asked, "Mommy, do they both have the same milk?"

"Yes," I answered.

Pointing to his own chest, he replied, "When I grow up, I will have one that tastes like vanilla, and the other will be chocolate!"

Marianne Shine

Santa's List

It's Christmas time again. As I hurry through the mall, I notice a line of children waiting to see Santa. The bearded man in red glances in my direction. I can tell he recognizes me as he scans the naughty and nice list he holds in his mittened hand. There's no mistake in which column he finds my name!

It all started a couple of years ago when our son was six months old. My husband and I wanted a special holiday picture of our new baby sitting on Santa's lap. "Let's go during the supper hour," I suggested to my husband. "There shouldn't be much of a line then."

The following evening, I dressed the baby in his fluffy blue jacket with the long bunny ears and headed for Memory Mall.

When my husband saw the long line of children, he groaned. "I thought no one would be here," he said.

"Looks like everyone had the same idea," I replied. "But one quick little picture shouldn't take too long."

We went to the end of the line and waited. When it was our turn, I climbed the steps to Santa's castle and walked over to where he sat in a large rocking chair. "We just want a picture," I said as I happily placed our little son on Santa's lap.

The elf in charge of pictures quickly snapped the shutter of her camera. Then she turned to me. "I'm finished. You can get the baby," she said.

I stepped forward, thinking Santa would hand the baby to me. He didn't. He just sat in his rocking chair with the baby on his lap. A moment or two passed, and still nothing happened.

The impatient eyes of all the little children were on me. Deciding to take matters, and the baby, into my own hands, I leaned down and put my arms around the fluffy blue bunny jacket. With the baby firmly in my grasp, I began lifting him to me.

Suddenly a deep voice boomed, "Lady... let go of my beard!"

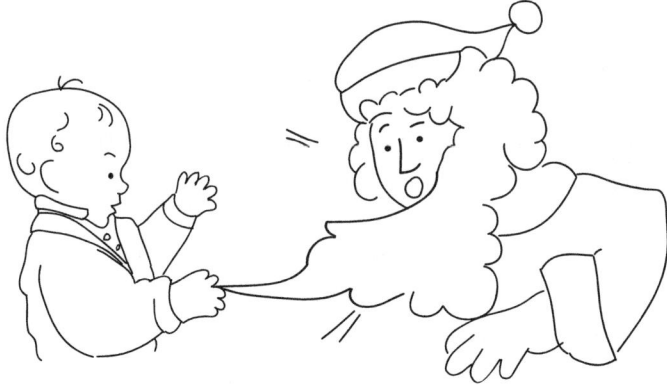

I looked at Santa. I froze. Somehow, his beard had been pulled at least six inches away from his face.

Santa cried out again. "Hey, lady...let go!"

To my horror, I realized I had accidentally grabbed Santa's beard along with the baby's fluffy jacket. Santa was yelling at ME!

Time stood still. From the corner of my eye, I saw the stunned expression on the elf's face. The eyes of all those children were on me...again! Frantically, I looked over to where my husband was standing. He just looked back at me and slowly shook his head.

Santa quickly brought me back to reality.

"Please...just let go of my beard!" I released it as quickly as I could. There was a very loud snapping sound followed by an even louder, "Ouch!"

"Oh, Santa," I began. "I didn't mean...."

"Just go, and leave me alone," Santa ordered. He rubbed his chin and glared at me.

Embarrassed, I scurried away with the baby to where my husband was waiting.

"It's not good to upset Santa," he pretended to scold. "We are sure to be at the top of Santa's list now... only it's the wrong one!"

Bonnie J. Shirley

Surprise Visitor

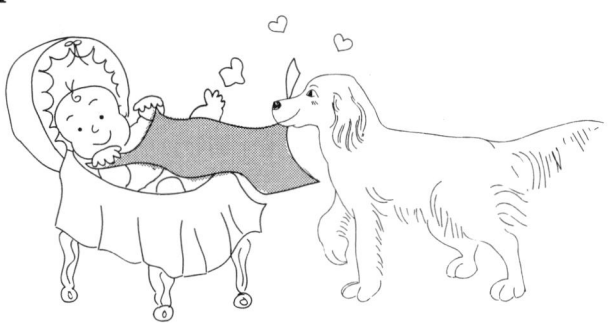

The birth of our first child prompted a kind phone call from the wife of my husband's employer. She wanted to stop by with a gift.

I tried to hide my shock when I opened the door and was greeted not only by the boss' wife, but also by an enormous Irish setter merrily wagging its tail.

The dog trotted in on the lady's heels and headed straight for the baby's basket. I was terrified that he would tip the basket over, or worse. Our visitor did not seem at all concerned about the dog's behavior as he continued bounding through our house.

I decided to trust the owner's instincts, but the short visit still seemed like an eternity.

"Can she tell how relieved I am?" I thought, as the lady stood to leave and the enthusiastic dog followed. She headed out the door while leaving the dog standing there, and I screeched as nicely as I could, "Don't forget your dog!"

"My dog?" she replied with a horrific look on her face, "I thought it was *your* dog. I wondered about such a big dog around your baby!"

Later that evening, our canine "visitor" was discovered to be a neighborhood pet. My boss' wife and I had many a belly laugh over our mishap. What we were both grateful for, though, was that the Irish Setter had the disposition of a lamb. He just wanted to welcome the neighborhood's newest addition!

Mary Jane Vernon

Let's Pretend

My grandson was unintentionally born at home in the living room. In the midst of the bedlam, the baby's four-year-old sister, Becca, and older sister, Courtney, were told to go to their bedroom.

Becca visits me often and likes me to play "house" with her. Usually she chooses to be the mommy and I'm the little girl. Not too long after the birth of her little brother, we were playing "house." The dialogue went something like this:

Becca: "Play like you didn't know I was going to have a baby."

Grammy: "Okay."

Becca: (As she's putting her doll underneath her blouse.) "Honey, Mommy's going to have a baby. Do you want to touch Mommy's tummy and feel it moving?"

Grammy: "Oh, Mommy, Mommy! I can feel it moving!" (Play acting.)

Becca: (Suddenly) "Okay, Mommy's going to have the baby now." (She climbs on the bed.)

Becca: (Groaning, long and drawn out.) "OOOOOOH, AAAAAAH, OHHHHH, UMMMMMM." (Fast breathing, groaning continues for quite some time, sounding exactly like a woman in hard labor)

Grammy: (In her regular grandma voice) "Becca, what are you doing?"

Becca: (Indignantly) "I'M HAVING A BABY!" (Continues with her labor.)

Grammy: "Why are you making all those noises?"

Becca:(Exasperated) "Be-cuzzz Gram-mee, that's what you have to do to have a Ba-bee!"

Becca: "There, (pulls doll from underneath blouse.) I've had the baby. (To me) Oh, honey, it's a girl! Honey, come see your new baby sister."

Grammy: (As Grammy) "Becca, how do you know so much about having a baby?"

Becca: "Because that's what Mommy was doing when she had Alex."

Grammy: "But I thought you and Courtney were in the bedroom."

Becca: (Matter-of-factly) "Yeah, but we peeked around the corner."

Nellie Grafke

Down In The Dumps

I was down in the dumps recently.

It all began when Joan phoned me at work. "Raymond's diapers are missing!" she cried. "The diaperman couldn't find the diaper bag. The garbage people probably picked it up. The diaperman said we have to pay $100 to replace the lost diapers. What're we going to do, Joe?"

The diapers and garbage are picked up within minutes of each other every Tuesday morning. It's been my responsibility, since we moved into our apartment last month, to take the bag of diapers downstairs and leave it behind the steel gate so it won't get mixed up with the garbage I leave in front of the gate.

"Someone in the building must have put the bag near the garbage," I said. "Why don't you call the garbage people to see if we can get the diapers back."

Ten minutes later Joan called back. "They found

the diapers! They said I can pick the bag up at the dump. Truck 6A will be waiting for me. Raymond's taking his nap and they told me to be there right away. What should I do?" she asked.

No wife and baby of mine are going to the dump. "I'll go," I said.

I zoomed down to the city dump and parked outside the gate. I was expecting to find truck 6A, pick up the diapers and hurry back to work. The man at the checkpoint said the truck was waiting for me up the hill and around the bend. As I started up the hill, a man in a green pickup truck, the supervisor, stopped and asked, "Are you the guy who's looking for the diapers?"

"Yeah," I said, feeling a little embarrassed. Diapers? Who cares about diapers? People rush to the dump to look for antiques or diamonds, not diapers.

The dump site was a cavernous structure. Two guys jumped out of truck 6A when the supervisor and I arrived. One guy was tall and solidly built, the other was short and lean. I was set to grab the diapers, thank the men and be on my way. But it wasn't to be.

"We'll empty the garbage here," said the supervisor, pointing to the cement floor we were standing on and not the enormous dump twenty feet below. "It'll cost you $100 to get someone to sweep the garbage into the dump."

"I'll sweep the garbage," I offered.

Tall and Short looked at each other and laughed.

"You don't know what you're saying," said the supervisor.

"But I don't have $100 on me. And now I don't even know if the diapers are in the truck."

"I'm pretty sure I picked up the diapers," said Short. "I couldn't figure out why someone would leave them for garbage."

"Can't you drop the load in the dump and I'll look for the bag down there?"

"No one's allowed down there," replied the supervisor adamantly, because "down there" was where garbage was really garbage. There were all kinds of things you could squish into, fall into, cut yourself with and God knows what else could happen. "Look," he said, "I'll charge the $100 to your garbage bill."

No matter what I did, I was out $100. I was struck dumb.

Sprinklers were spraying water lightly from the tall ceiling above. It was dusty, dirty, dank, and the smell, oh, the smell– it was the city dump! And the noise level made it almost impossible to think, what with an endless flow of trucks driving in, emptying their loads and driving out and two huge Caterpillar tractors going back and forth leveling the garbage.

"Come on," I overheard Tall say to Short, "it won't take long."

"You help the guy," griped Short. "We've been up since three in the morning. I'm pooped."

"Then I'll help the guy myself," said Tall.

"You win," said Short, and he looked at the supervisor. "Forget the $100."

It's nice of these guys to help out, I thought, but why are they making such a big deal out of sweeping up some garbage?

The plan was to let a little garbage out at a time and check for the diaper bag. Short tilted the truckbed back and moved the truck forward as Tall and I searched for the white plastic bag. No dice. A second load was let out. Nothing. A third load–that's when Tall spied the white plastic bag of diapers.

The next order of business was to get the garbage into the dump. It was piled three feet high and covered an area equivalent to a medium-sized bedroom. Each of us had a shovel and we began chopping into the sides of the pile and scraping it into the dump. That's when I realized why Tall and Short had their little disagreement. The garbage was like lead and it took every ounce of energy to move that ooey, gooey, smelly garbage into the dump. I was huffing and puffing, groaning and sweating and didn't let up for one second. I wanted to show those two men (I never did get their names) how indebted I was to them by working doubly fast so as to lighten their load a bit. If it weren't for me, they would've been home with a beer in hand.

It took an hour to get the garbage into the dump. I was totally exhausted. I offered Tall and Short all the money I had, $30.00, but they declined.

What kind of people are these garbage guys? I wondered.

I grabbed Raymond's diapers and was about to race back to my car, when Tall offered me a ride in his truck. After he dropped me off, I said, "You guys are saints. That's what you are — true saints. I'm going to leave you guys some cold beer next week, and all the weeks after that, too."

"Forget the beer," he smiled. "Any kind of soft drink'll do fine."

That's the story of how one man's trash became three men's buried treasure. And that is the last time little Raymond is going to get me "down in the dumps!"

Joe Sutton

Our House

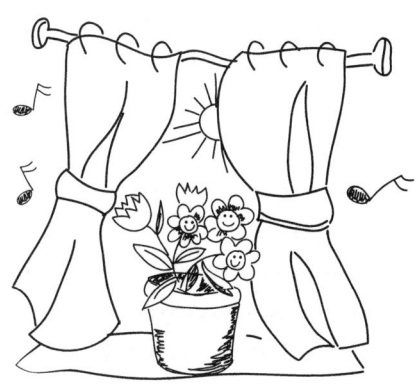

We built a new house three years ago. Watched it being built from the concrete piers to the textured paint and glazed tile. It was a new couple's house, with vaulted ceilings, bay windows and carpet a color called champagne toast. We paid attention to detail; Riverside Shakespeare and oversized art books under the glass coffee table, one cobalt blue vase on the fireplace ledge, plants with vines traveling from ceiling to floor.

Our house wore the first two years well. But this third year has been a different story. Shower curtains now protect the "champagne toast" carpet beneath two highchairs. The rest has been tie-dyed various shades of Juicy Juice. The bottom three slats on each venetian blind are bent towards heaven. There is tupperware in the toy cabinet and there are toys in the tupperware drawer. Cheerios adorn table tops, window sills and throw rugs. One tiny blue shoe sits in the hallway.

On top of the fireplace mantel are matches, screws, coins, coffee cups, coke cans, pencils, pens and stacks of diapers! Lint covered binkies lie between the couch cushions. The floor is covered with blocks, Tonka trucks, a fire engine, two tyke bikes and a train.

Every board book has a bite taken out of it. There is a comforter over the fireplace ledge, a playpen in front of the electrical outlet and no plant lives below the five foot mark. The glass coffee table now brandishes sticky hand prints and opaque milk rings from abandoned baby bottles. The T.V. remote is missing in action. The springs on the doorstops have been removed. The door to the stereo unit hangs by a hinge. A chair leans up against it.

In the living room, one twin boy turns circles to Barney's theme song…"I love you, you love me…" The other little boy skips around the couch with a Winnie the Pooh sheet over his head. They collide and giggle. And I think, what one year can do to the value of a home!

Laura Stavoe Harm

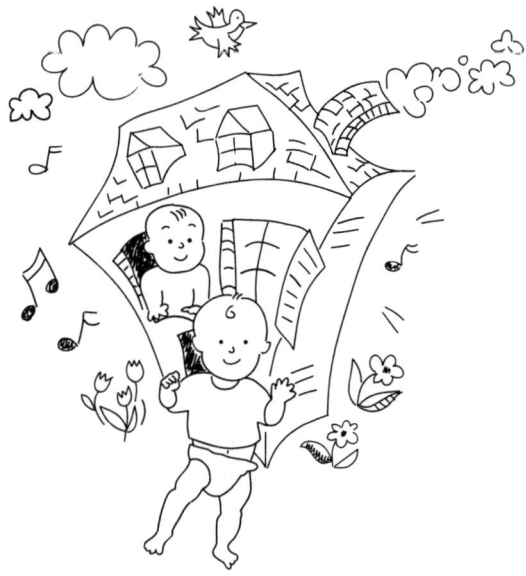

Little Miss Know-It-All

Our parents threw us a baby shower in January 1999. I was seven months pregnant and nothing but belly. Three of my young nieces were helping me open gifts, which I held up to show everyone. A couple of gifts were really too large for a very pregnant lady to lift, but not wanting to offend the giver, I lifted them up anyway.

My sister-in-law was worried about my efforts. She said, "You better stop lifting those big gifts or that baby is going to come out right now."

My seven-year-old niece, Alé, looked me up and down. Then she said in an authoritative voice, "Well, it won't go very far. *She's wearing pantyhose!*"

Valerie L. Fred

Dog Days

My wife left me at home one evening with our four-month-old daughter. That was a first. Not long after her departure, I entered the baby's room and was immediately confronted with a decided shift in odors. I knew we were in trouble.

I quickly dialed both grandmothers. No answer. I

tried my aunt next door, and my sister, too. No one was home. I was hopelessly trapped.

I realized what I must do. As I held my breath, I laid my daughter on the bed and removed the poopy diaper. I tossed it on the floor behind me and went to get a wet washcloth.

When I returned, things went from bad to worse! As I struggled to tackle the task-at-hand, I heard a strange sound behind me.

Our canine garbage disposal, Sherman, had wandered into the room and was feasting on the dirty diaper. Uhhhhggggg!

Nature, though, soon disagreed with Sherman's choice of entrees and things erupted before my very eyes. My lunch, too, was soon defying gravity. What a sorry sight we were!

Needless to say, from then on, I reserved the right to change only "wet" diapers. I guess there are a few things only moms have the stomach for.

Doug Huston

Caution! Explosive!

Thank goodness for a sense of humor. Pregnancy with twins is a s-t-r-e-t-c-h-i-n-g experience anyway, and this comment added a bright spot during my expansive last few months:

Upon walking in on me in a stage of undress, my daughter exclaimed, "Mama, your belly button is EXPLODING!"

as told to Lori Perdew

Chapter 5

Delivery Dilemmas

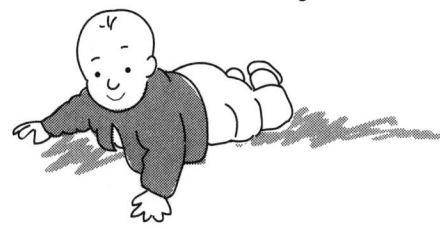

Born at the Slurpee Machine?

A little misunderstanding can become a treasured piece of personal history.

My sister called with the news. Since neither my husband or I was home, she talked to our son, Kevin.

"Hi, Kevin, Julie's twins were born this morning," Aunt Harriet said. "At 7-11!"

"Wow, that must have been pretty traumatic," he said, while his mind envisioned babies being born around the Slurpee machine.

Julie is his first cousin, my niece.

"Yes," Harriet said. "They were just short of thirty-one weeks along!"

"Gee... that sounds serious, how are they doing?" he inquired.

"They each weighed over three pounds — both boys. And they're stable. We'll keep you posted." Harriet added.

So that evening when we talked to Kevin he told us we better call Harriet, and quick!

"She sounded pretty frazzled. Julie had her babies two months prematurely at 7-11. I've let everyone know!" Kevin said with concern in his voice.

I dreaded dialing her number.

The tile floors, bread racks and drafty coolers of the convenience store flashed through my mind. What an awful experience it must have been for my poor niece! This was not the setting to effectively handle premature newborns. What were their chances?

Finally I worked up the courage to call my sister, the new Grandma.

"Kevin said the babies came?" I ventured, when Harriet picked up the phone.

"Yes, they are both on respirators, but doing fine," she said.

"So... they were born this morning?" I gingerly asked, preparing myself for the wild escapade.

"Julie went into labor a couple days ago, and they admitted her and tried to stop it, but it didn't work," she continued. "We're just lucky she was at the best neo-natal hospital this side of the Mayo Clinic. Anyway, they were finally born this morning: Teague at 7:11, and Tucker at 7:12."

I breathed a sigh of relief, chuckled quietly and didn't interrupt the details that followed to share our own twisted version of this blessed event. Someday I will. And it will become part of the legacy of the twins' birth — a tiny nugget of personal history to be polished by telling and retelling.

Driving by the 7-11 always brings a smile to my face as I recall our little family mis-communication. It also brings warm thoughts of the miracle of birth, not to mention the anticipation of taking my grand nephews for their very first Slurpee!

Joyce Rabas
excerpted, The Sun Newspaper, 1998

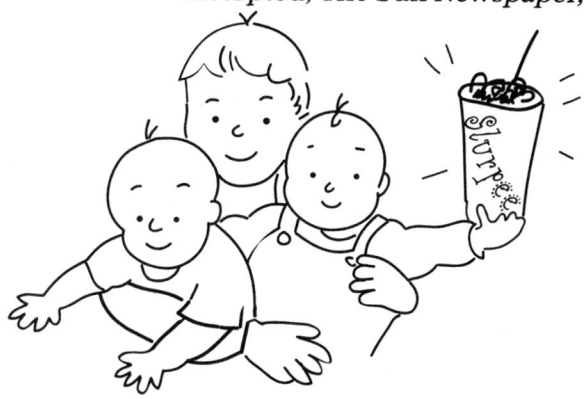

Coach Dad Pinch Hits

I'm a grandfather. That's something nice that can happen to one who lives long enough.

My journey to grandparenting took some curious turns. It started when my daughter Mary-Kim and her husband decided she should move back in with Mom and Dad. She planned to complete her school teaching year before joining her husband in their new Southern home.

Then my daughter posed a question. "Dad, would you be my natural childbirth coach?" She explained that since my wife, Adele, traveled a great deal in her job, she was frequently inaccessible. As a high school teacher, I remained anchored to a home base.

I blurted out, "How about your husband, Steve?"

"The baby's due during the basketball season. Since he's a coach, chances are he'll be on the road," she said.

The logic seemed sound. My son-in-law traveled to several cities a month. He couldn't serve as a childbirth coach, too. Not from thousands of miles away. My excited daughter said, "Dad, you did it when my little brother, Jon, was born. You were a pioneer then. Just take a refresher course."

Excitement slowly displaced the trace of horror camped in my gut. "Sure," I said with bravado. "I'll be glad to help."

The next day, waiting room stares accompanied my visit to the gynecologist. It seemed that the half dozen clients and spouses in the waiting room scrutinized Mary-Kim and me with a collective raised brow. Was my salty beard the problem? The three seated men reminded me of players on my last Little League team.

The receptionist called, "Mr. and Mrs. S, please come in."

"That's not my name," I mumbled as she ushered my daughter toward the scale.

"Step on this!" she ordered. So much for correcting the record.

The lady in white then squeezed us into a room no larger than a small outdoor tool shed. A shoeless shoe rack dangled from the door. Instead of footwear, booklets leaned out with titles such as *"Fertility Problems," "Making Your Changing Years Better"* and *"Positive Healing."*

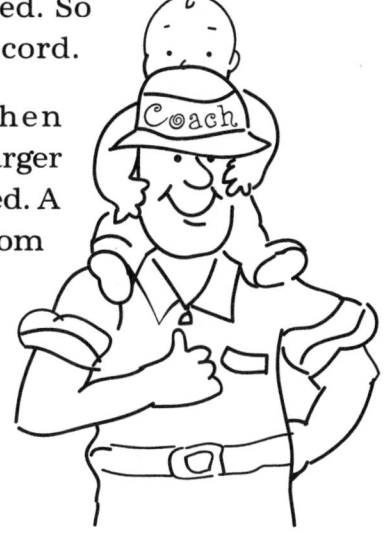

Directly above the paper-cloaked examination table hovered several plastic gulls. I made them spin. Someone entered the room. She raised her eyes toward the performing gulls and smiled.

"Doc," my daughter said, "this is my dad."

Times change. This doctor looked more like an Olympic gymnast than a woman of medicine. The doctor said, "He doesn't look old enough." That insightful observation fueled my ego.

The doctor attached a space-aged device called a fetal monitor to the expectant mother. A tiny flashing heart winked at me. I heard my grandchild's heartbeat in quadraphonic stereo. The doctor added, "Put on a good show for Grandpa, kid. This could be worth big bucks." I felt confident, I passed my first coaching test.

The next day, I visited the library. Shelves of books describing natural childbirth faced me. I yanked some. I discovered that books written about Grandpa as coach are nonexistent. I studied the books. I understood breathing. I knew all about the contractions of childbirth. Time for my big test. I felt prepared.

A week before my scheduled classes, I learned about the conspiracy. My wife and daughter planned to gently dismiss me from the coaching job. I made it easy for them and resigned the night before class. I said, "You two go without me. It's better as a mother-daughter thing." I was glad they agreed, but disappointed they failed to protest.

Mom and daughter bonded. They attended class together. They shared late night tea. They spoke of contractions, breathing and baby room decorations. I accepted my dismissal with class.

A week before the due date, Steve flew home for a brief visit. A few days later, he flew halfway around the country for a road game. On that crisp Friday morn, I accepted the assignment of driving him over the glistening, crackling ice to the local airport. Several hours later, I traveled the same, now slushy road taking my daughter to the doctor.

At the doctor's office, the nurse ordered Mary-Kim to lie down. The same stereo attachments I'd seen before were plugged and pasted around her tummy. The baby's heartbeat resounded. But I sensed a problem knitted in the nurse's brow as she watched the numbers.

A harried nurse disconnected the monitor and whisked us to a room upstairs. This time, sonar equipment resembling submarine paraphernalia was attached to the expectant mother. The screen televised the baby. On the wall hung a chart depicting male and female babies. I studied the diagrams. I solved the puzzle. Obviously, my daughter carried my grandson.

We returned to the reception area to await instructions. The nurse scurried out, grabbed my daughter's hand, and blurted, "Mrs. S, the doctor wants to give you an internal. Immediately!"

Ten minutes later, my daughter returned. "Granddad," she said, "we're going to the hospital."

"No, you don't understand," I pleaded. "Steve's not here. This is just a routine physical."

"I've lost amniotic fluid. We're going to induce."

I was a veteran. My middle child, Peter, was induced. But that happened way back when people took giant steps for mankind on the moon. Moisture dripped from my brow. The original script never included this. I opened the car door, and helped Mary-Kim in.

"Dad," she said, "I'm a little scared."

A little scared. My body quivered. We needed her mom, my wife, Adele, at this critical moment. I mustered courage. "Don't worry. I've been through this before, with your mom. Before long my little girl will have her own baby." I wiped and kissed her brow.

The hospital expected us. An attendant greeted us at the entrance and led us into a special room. The VIP treatment prevailed until we faced some forms, related to record release, health insurance and assorted other topics. My daughter balked at the final form.

"What about this one?"

"That's so we can give you blood should you require it."

"That won't be needed. My dad is a universal donor."

I squirmed. I looked at my left bicep. I glared at my chatty child. Color drained from my skin. My own flesh and blood gave me up. She offered her hypochondriac father as a human sacrifice.

I remained stoic. I wondered, when did I become a player? I signed on as a substitute coach. I now served as a substitute, substitute coach. The nurse tersely said, "Sorry, can't use Dad. Blood has to be here a week."

"You're off the hook, Dad," my infidel said. "Guess you're coach again."

I excused myself and jogged toward the nearest phone.

I called home. No answer. I then called both Adele's office and her beeper. No answer. I rushed back to my daughter.

The reality of the delivery room jolted me. Immersed in the Coach Dad spirit, I prepared to offer my expertise. My child needed me more than ever. The old pro in Dad would not fail her. The delivery nurse said, "Mr. S, we'll dress her and then give you the clothes to take to your car. Then come back immediately to help." I gave up my fight on the Mr. S name.

I was back in the game. I must have leaped and jumped toward the elevator. I pumped the down button a dozen times. Later, my daughter said, "I told the nurse you're my dad, not Mr. S." She answered, "Dad looked like a nervous Peter Pan. He dropped your bag of clothes all over the elevator." They both laughed.

I continued my dash toward my car, vaulting small snow banks. "Coach Dad" lived again. Mary-Kim needed him.

Winded, I huffed into the waiting room. My wife's greeting startled me. Disappointment and relief slowed my walk. My coaching days ended. I briefed Adele on the natal news, and wistfully watched her take the elevator.

Head drooping, I drove home to await the good news.

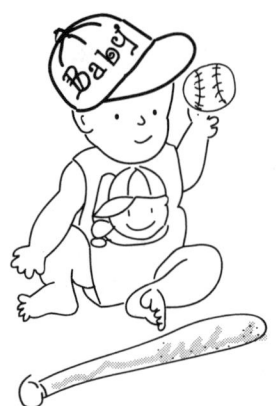

Three hours later, Coach Mom returned to the sidelines, too. Steve, the official head coach in this arena, flew back from his game. A few minutes after his return, my granddaughter Alee was born. So much, too, for my expertise as a baby handicapper. I predicted a boy.

My return to the coaching ranks of natural childbirth proved short-lived. Somehow all that mattered was this vibrant granddaughter who looked exactly like Granddad.

F. Anthony D'Alessandro

Cold Night, Warm Memory

It was a little before midnight when the pains began.

"They couldn't be labor pains, honey," I explained to my wife. "You're not due yet. And besides, these pains don't fit the patterns we were taught in Lamaze. Remember your labor pains with Dawn? Nothing like what you're having now. Right?"

I was calm, reasonable and reassuring. Somehow ,

my calmness and reassurance didn't make it all the way from my mouth to her ears.

"Call the doctor...now!" was all she said. And because of the way she said it, I sensed it was not a good time to discuss the matter any further. Better to wake the doctor at midnight than to continue walking down this lonely and dangerous path.

The doctor responded quickly to my call. False labor, he determined. His advice for her was to take a warm bath, get a good night's sleep and come to the hospital first thing in the morning. I felt vindicated.

"False labor," I said with confidence to my wife. "Take a warm bath, get a good night's sleep and we'll go to the hospital tomorrow morning."

Hearing this while curled in a fetal position on our bed, my wife took on a countenance that caused me to begin perspiring, even though it was a cold, March night.

"I'll get your bath ready," I said, hoping this would appease whatever it was that had suddenly taken possession of my wife. Three minutes into the bath the pains began again, only with more intensity. My wife reached out to me. I'm not sure whether it was for help or if she was trying to get a hand on my throat.

She spoke. *"Call him back. Tell him this is real labor and there will be no good night's sleep for any of us tonight!"*

There is a certain peace in being with a woman in labor. Under normal circumstances, men are cognitive creatures, attempting always to apply reason and rationality to any given situation. But when a man is with a woman in labor, he surrenders millions of years of genetic programming and becomes what's necessary for his near-term survival — a mindless idiot. He does only what is commanded of him and generates no thinking on his own.

I placed the call.

I informed the doctor we were on our way, woke our daughter, took her to the neighbor's house and returned to help my wife and her bag into our new car.

I thought about what might happen to the cloth seatcovers if her water should happen to break. But understanding I was still an idiot, I let the thought pass. I hopped in and we began our race to the hospital. During the day, the trip might take forty minutes. But at midnight, with light traffic and a liberal interpretation of speed limit signs, I figured I could make it in twenty. My wife's intensifying and more frequent contractions convinced me eighteen would be even better.

I was concentrating on my driving, when suddenly my right arm exploded in pain. I've been shot, I thought to myself. I instinctively tried to jerk my arm away, to the left, but it would not move. Oh, Geez — I'm paralyzed, too! With frightened hesitation, I looked at my arm. My wife was clutching it with her left hand. If I hadn't been wearing a leather jacket, I believe her fingers would have been pressed through my flesh and bone until they connected with the flesh of her own palm.

"Shall we try our Lamaze breathing?" I asked.

Her body went straight as a board — heels on the floorboards and neck supported by the headrest. I thought she was beginning to levitate. With the combined voices of a thousand demons rising from the deepest, most hellish part of her soul, all she said was, "Get there." I drove on, grappling with the thought of how life was going to be without the use of my right arm.

We arrived and I found a parking spot fairly close to the front entrance. Lamaze taught us to use the main entrance. The emergency room, after all, was for emergencies only.

I helped her from the car. With her bag in my nearly useless right hand and my left arm around her waist, we began the short walk to the hospital's front doors.

It was then her water broke. "The baby's coming!" she cried.

"No, no, that can't be because — uh — you see — we're not there yet." My observations didn't change her perceptions one bit. "The baby is coming out NOW!" she screamed. I was beginning to panic.

I hoisted her onto my hip and struggled to the sidewalk near the main entrance. "The baby IS COMING NOW!" she cried again. I laid her and her bag on the sidewalk and ran to the front doors. — Locked! I pounded on the doors and screamed, "My wife's having a baby out here! Come quick!"

I ran back to her, making a mental note to send a strongly worded letter to the Lamaze folks once I got home. She was on her back and I took a look. Indeed, the top of the baby's head was visible. Still no response from inside the hospital.

Suddenly, everything seemed very quiet and peaceful. I felt serene and calm. There were no more options, no choices, no more rushing. I was not aware of the night, the cold, the sidewalk, the street noise, or the light snow which was beginning to fall. I was aware only of my wife and the imminent birth. The only thing to do was to have the baby — there and then.

The baby made the transition from my wife's womb to my hands as naturally as a football passes from a center to his quarterback. The warmth of the baby's body meeting the cold, night air caused a curious steam to rise. Breathing? I couldn't tell. Not much light. What about the umbilical cord? Was it around the neck? I felt with my fingers. No, the neck was clear. But no breathing! What to do? Mouth-to-mouth! No, wait — a smack on the butt. 'Doc' Adams on *Gunsmoke* did it plenty of times!

I swung the baby by the ankles and was ready to deliver the blow that I prayed would work. I didn't have to. The swing upside down was all it took. Our new baby girl was breathing on her own.

"It's a girl," I whispered as I lay her down with my wife, who smiled. Watch check — 1:03 a.m., March 30.

I was snapped back to the world as the hospital entrance lights went on. Medical personnel with supplies and a gurney descended upon us. I stepped aside while they quickly checked both the baby and my wife, placed them on the gurney and rushed inside.

"Everything looks great," I heard someone say as the entourage entered the building and rounded a corner out of sight. I paused a moment, picked up the bag and followed.

Now fifteen years later, my memories and feelings of that night are vivid and mixed. Thank God we made it and thank God the hospital personnel were there to help. But also, thank God for the experience — the delivery on the sidewalk, the first breath, the curious steam mixing with the lightly falling snow on that beautiful and incredible night. I felt both relief and sadness when the lights came on and the people came to rescue us.

Our once-in-a-lifetime, magnificent, magical moment was over.

James Schirmer

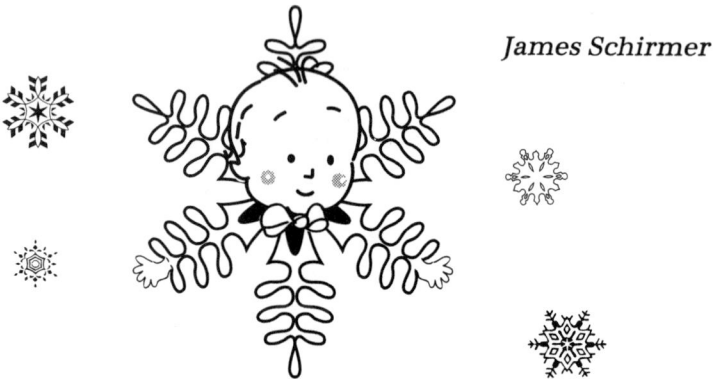

Baby on Deck

The birth of Barbara McGlynn's third child was as natural and as American as baseball. May 4, 1976. A cold spring day. The bottom of the ninth, and the game had moved into extra innings.

8 a.m.

Barbara notes that baby on deck is one week overdue, apparently happy to continue life out of the spotlight's glare.

11 a.m.

Barbara consults with her obstetrician, who dismisses her desperate, "When will this baby come?" with a cheerful, "A ripe apple will fall." Less than satisfied and wishing her jovial doctor could shoulder some of her load instead of offering her a cliché-ridden pep talk, Barbara shuffles home. As morning drags into afternoon, she makes a valiant effort to keep up with some energetic rookies, three and six years old, in the dugout. She vows to hang up her spikes at the end of this season.

5 p.m.

Barb struggles to make supper, but with a nagging backache, she just can't swing it. She tells her family to fend for themselves. Hot dogs, cotton candy, soda, peanuts. She couldn't care less.

Her husband, Dick, offers to help. Barb thanks him for his team spirit but observes that if he can't *have* this baby, his value to her is limited. Hoping to relax, Barb heads for her bed, but the pressure, both physical and psychological, begins to mount.

7 p.m.

"You want to renegotiate contractions?" baby on deck asks Barb, who immediately packs her bag for the hospital. The children watch television while Barb struggles into the passenger seat of the family car. Baby on deck decides that a home birth is preferable to the drugged-up comfort of 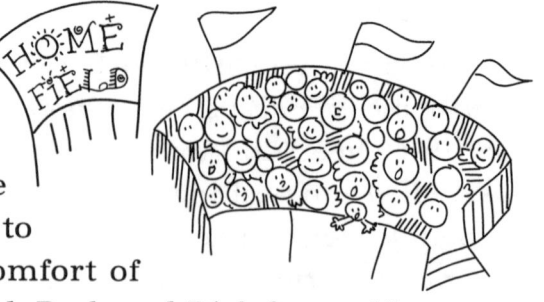 the maternity ward. Barb and Dick face a dilemma: Should they try to make it back into the house or allow baby on deck to call the plays? The decision is made when Barb discovers she is unable to reclimb the stairs.

She crawls into the car's back seat. Her panicked husband calls 911 for some backup.

"Don't move until the ambulance gets here!" Dick tells Barb.

Moments later, baby shows his father who's got star billing by crowning into view beneath the streetlight that illuminates the driveway as if it were a stadium. With Barb's third push, Dick performs the role of catcher at home plate.

"Strike three. You're out. It's a boy! We won!" Dick says. He waves the baby over Barb like a pennant. She nods off, but not before imagining the appreciative roar of a crowd.

She awakens to hear the ambulance attendants, (who spent time at the wrong house) debating their transfer method. The attendants decide a board will suffice. Barb feels as if she's just been moved from the comfort of the front office to the bullpen. She grimaces all the way to the hospital.

The staff doctors and nurses in the ER proclaim Dick the hero of the hour, brushing off Barb as a minor league player. Full of bravado, Dick demands a refund for half the obstetrician's fee. The doctor merely chuckles, pats Barb's knee and declares, "The ripe apple has fallen."

Barb makes a mental note to tell Dick to find a better agent. Later she will joke about her baby on deck, baby on board, and how there's nothing minor league about pitching a winner— a nine-pound, three-ounce boy. She and Dick will announce an agreement to terms the following summer. Barb will not retire. She will be pregnant with their fourth child.

Jennifer Litt

Deliver Me From Due Dates

My obstetricians have always been lovely people. But I have the sneaking suspicion that when it comes to estimating due dates and other phenomena, they poke, measure and monitor, then retreat to their office sanctuaries to throw one set of dice marked January through December and another marked one through thirty-one.

I formed this theory while pregnant with my first child. A bride of a mere six weeks, I reported to my husband that I was three days overdue and might be pregnant. Hubby reminded me that he had used "something" and I had used "something," and therefore there was absolutely no chance I was expecting "anything."

Three weeks later I convinced him to take me to our local clinic for testing. My impending motherhood was confirmed.

I made an appointment with a very eminent obstetrician. He examined me thoroughly. Afterward he informed me, in patriarchal tones, that I was three months pregnant according to the color of my innards and the baby was due at Thanksgiving. I went home and cried.

But I adjusted, as people do. I knitted. I went to second-hand shops for baby things. I went to the obstetrician once a month, a long bus ride clear across town.

At my September visit the doctor looked concerned.

"This baby's pretty big," he said. "It looks like it might come earlier than expected."

In October, I began weekly visits for pelvic exams to check on my progress. October passed; November passed. I seemed to spend my entire life on that long bus ride to and from the doctor's office. Each time the doctor cheerfully said, "Any time now."

December came. I looked like a walrus. My mother, ever hopeful, traveled 400 miles to take care of me and the baby when I came home from the hospital.

I made yet another visit to the obstetrician's office. The nurse looked at me kind of funny and said, jokingly she thought, "Are you still around?" The doctor also looked at me kind of funny, was silent a moment, then said, "Any time now."

By December 31, I had perfected sobbing to a fine art. I ate prunes. I ate figs. I drank lots of orange juice. I took a five-mile waddle. I jumped up and down on the double bed of our apartment and broke the slats. The spinster lady chided me for doing "that type of thing" so enthusiastically in my current condition. My mother went home.

January 12. Another weekly visit to the doctor. This time a worried frown creased his forehead. "It's a real big baby," he said.

"Is it ever going to be born?" I asked.

"You're not the least bit dilated," he replied. "Might be another week."

I went into labor that night.

Rachel was seven-pounds, five-ounces, a skinny, long-legged smidge of a kid. While I was recuperating, I calculated that I had gotten pregnant after the bunny said "positive" and after I had thrown out my "something" and my spouse his "something." When I was ready for such diversions again, I used a different type of contraceptive.

Almost precisely two years later, I again informed my spouse that I thought I was pregnant. We were in the Army, living in a converted restaurant in very rural Europe. My spouse's response was, "Impossible." He reminded me that we had always been very careful about using . . .

The military obstetrician informed me I was three months pregnant, if not more. I told him about my prior adventure. He said, "I assure you, I know what I'm talking about."

We arrived stateside when I was eight months pregnant. The renowned civilian obstetrician whom I consulted said "any day now." He also said I had a very narrow pelvis and it was lucky this was a small baby so I wouldn't have to have a Cesarean delivery.

Karen was almost three weeks overdue. After my entrance examination at the hospital, the doctor said I had hours to go, told me again not to worry because it was a small baby, then went out to breakfast with my spouse.

A half-hour later the nurse did a cursory examination and then zap...onto the delivery table. The doctor didn't even get to finish his scrambled eggs. The baby weighed nine-pounds, three-ounces.

I went home and tried a different type of contraceptive. The "loop" was still in place a year and a half later when the group medical plan physician informed me I was pregnant. He took the loop out and gave it to me as a souvenir. "At least this one will be a boy," he consoled.

Laura was two weeks late, arriving during my obstetrician's annual vacation. He told me he had planned his vacation for that date because he knew the baby would have already arrived and he wouldn't have to worry about me.

By then I had become something of a skeptic. But at least I didn't have to worry about any more kids. I had developed some type of female problem that caused a different obstetrician to inform me I was sterile. That diagnosis is on my records someplace. It was still there six years later, when I told the obstetrician I was pregnant.

"Impossible," he said.

Sally was two weeks late. On my last visit to the obstetrician I was so neurotic I asked him to induce labor. "You're not due for at least three weeks," he said. "There's not a sign of dilation."

I went into labor three hours after I returned home.

Sally is a great kid. Laura, Karen and Rachel are great kids, too.

I had my tubes tied.

Pat Kite

The Lopata Way

When I was a child, my family traveled every year. And we always had adventures. Miss a plane? Lose baggage? Hotels closed? It was, as we called it, "The Lopata Way." I should have known that when I went to Ukraine and Russia to adopt a baby, I'd go the Lopata Way.

In the winter of 1993 my husband, Paul, and I received word of a baby girl awaiting adoption in Simferopol, Ukraine. We got out the atlas to see where we were going and spent months practicing saying "Sim-fer-o-pol." By the time we figured out how to pronounce it, it was June and we were ready to go.

Our trip began the Lopata Way, with a tedious two-hour drive to Boston and the world's only airport connected to the rest of humanity by a two-lane, perpetually blocked tunnel. The next fun was the seven-hour flight to Frankfurt, Germany. Gabriel, our three-year-old, cruised the aisles and put his tray table up and down about seven million times. He finally fell asleep, curled up in the window seat, during our next flight to Moscow.

The final leg of our journey was a two-day train ride to Simferopol. Our chaperone was Gennady, an affable Russian who spoke little English. He warned us to stay in first class and not wander about the train. I wish he could've explained the mysterious, late-night stops in the middle of nowhere. With loudspeakers blasting something in Russian and giant searchlights swinging around, we got the distinct sense we were on a cattle car headed to the gulag.

We finally arrived in Simferopol, a city about as exciting as interstate driving. Thank goodness our hosts for our three-week stay had four televisions (in their one-bedroom apartment) that we could watch and not understand a thing.

We soon succumbed to what the Russians called "going crazy in Russia," a common sickness that happens to Westerners who spend more than two weeks there.

Russia and Ukraine are not Western countries. They are not Eastern, either. They seem to have inherited the worst of both hemispheres. For instance, "manana" is supposedly a Latin American phenomenon. Nonsense. The Russians invented it and call it "Dun Worry." Your plane is leaving in fifteen minutes and

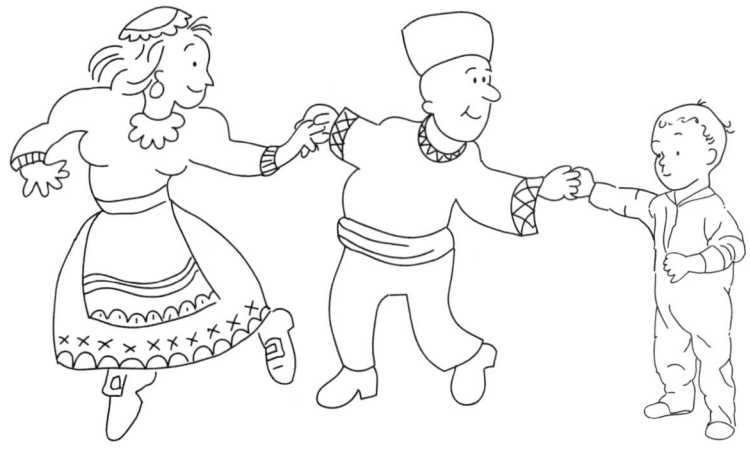

the airport is an hour away? "Dun Worry." Of course, Russians know that no planes leave within twelve hours of scheduled departure time anyway. Schedule? There's no direct translation in Russian.

The Russians, though, are forever kind, especially to children. They seem to love children more than anything.

For example, Simferopolitans, despite their poverty, are rich in playgrounds, many of which have amusement park rides that cost pennies to go on. Food is barely affordable, but a trip on the ferris wheel is. The Russians are also eager to help you with your children. Our son couldn't join us in court for our adoption proceedings, but the clerks kept him entertained. His eyes grew wide with fear, however, when grabby grandmas pulled him onto their laps so he would have a seat on the trolleys. They take seriously the adage that children belong to everyone.

Our stay in Simferopol was unexpectedly extended, so we did some sightseeing. We rode the longest trolley line in the world to Yalta, a resort town on the "Russian Riviera." We sat uncomfortable on a rock-strewn beach, watching Gabe frolic, wondering how he could be having such a good time. Throughout our travels he was unaffected by the greasy food, noxious city air and overgrown lawns.

Our grand finale toward home started with racing across the tarmac in Simferopol to board our plane back to Moscow, using Gabe in his stroller as offensive lineman, then battling with Russians and Germans for three seats together.

After takeoff our newly adopted daughter slept. Gabe wandered the aisles, and we watched numerous safety regulations being violated. Some people smoked, some stood by the airplane door to ensure a quick exit, some actually sat down. The aisles were overflowing with baggage, food and children. By the time we realized the food service was grab-what-you-can-get style, they'd run out. We snacked on crumbly American granola bars.

At the Moscow airport, where the temperature hovered around forty degrees, we shivered in our sandals and short sleeves. We huddled in blankets, looking like refugees, including the crying baby. Our driver pulled up in his two-door Fiat. For us? Of course. "Dun worry." We all squeezed into the backseat and luggage filled every other space.

Not too far down the road the car had a flat. "Dun worry" we thought. We all got out and waited, children in arms, for the driver to change the tire. Instead, at midnight, on a fairly deserted road, he stood in the middle of the road waving his arm.

Paul inquired, "Can I help change the tire?" The driver looked perplexed. "Tire? Tire? No tire." Ah, the familiar Lopata Way. The driver continued waving, turning to us occasionally to flash a smile and say,

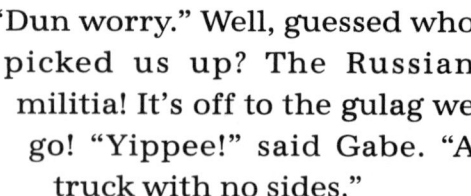

"Dun worry." Well, guessed who picked us up? The Russian militia! It's off to the gulag we go! "Yippee!" said Gabe. "A truck with no sides."

The militiamen dropped us off at what looked like a tenement in the South Bronx. We paid the soldiers for the ride in an extremely valuable currency — Snickers bars.

Our next exciting ride was in a pitch-black elevator. What fun! Though it was well after midnight when we arrived at the apartment, Gabe was as wide awake as a bat. Paul and I were ready for the last rites.

Despite all the "adventures," it was, of course, worth it. I developed some good thigh muscles using the holes they call toilets. We got a daughter, and our son got a sister. They fight like siblings everywhere. But instead of threatening to send her to Siberia like my big brothers did when I was little, Gabe threatens to take her back to Simferopol. Maybe someday they will go there together — the Lopata Way, of course.

Peg Lopata

Stork 747

It was a retired homicide detective, not an attending physician, who delivered my fiancee's new niece.

Of course, when the stork is a Boeing 747, the delivery room is Lambert Field in St. Louis and the parents have been expecting for more than a year and a half, anything can happen.

"Is there some celebrity on this plane?" a puzzled woman asked as we stood at the terminal gate.

She was eyeing our entourage, wondering if we were groupies with our stuffed bears, helium balloons and cameras snapping pictures nonstop. Behind the camcorder documenting every move, I jockeyed for position as if I were Steven Spielberg.

"Celebrity? Yes!" my fiancee's mother replied. "It's my new baby granddaughter from Korea."

Meanwhile, the expectant parents inched closer to the gate. Impatient as Larry and Robin were to meet their baby for the first time, they also were accustomed to waiting. Adoptive parents have to be.

They'd waited nineteen months and two days from the date they'd first attended a workshop on international adoption. After that meeting — and after more than twenty years of marriage — they made a commitment "to do what it takes" to adopt. So they'd waited to receive materials from more than twenty-five adoption agencies. Each agency and each country have requirements for adoptive parents; they learned they were automatically disqualified by some because they'd both reached forty. Other agencies proved beyond their financial reach, even though they were willing to part with every nickel of their life savings.

Choosing an international company, they applied for a Korean baby girl. And waited again, although their wait was far from idle. The paperwork was endless. Larry remembers making ninety copies of forms in one day. There were references to get. Fingerprinting to be done. Notaries to locate. Reams of information to read.

They attended adoptive parenting classes, and they learned about Korean culture through meetings of International Families. Caring friends and family members kept asking, "Is she here yet?" but they knew the child that would one day be theirs hadn't even been born. They had to wait.

One year and four months dragged by before they received a call at Christmastime that a baby was available. The agency forwarded photographs, a video and medical records for their pediatrician detailing a herniated umbilical cord the size of a lemon. Was this the right child for them? The agency asked.

Yes, yes, yes they answered, this is our baby. It

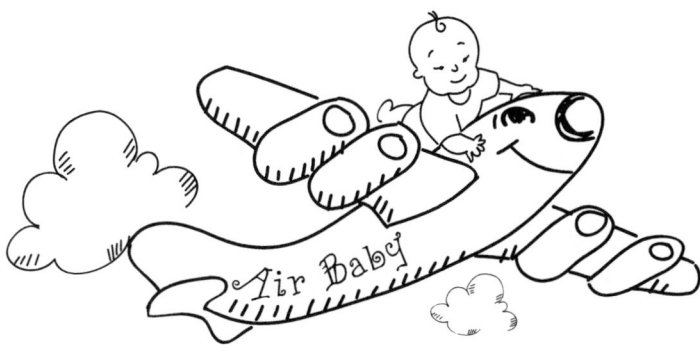

became a silent mantra as they painted her room bubblegum pink, wallpapered with pastel angels, bought furniture, researched the safest car seat. Surprise showers yielded necessities galore, including thirty-eight pairs of socks. Still they had to wait twelve more weeks for her arrival.

They got to the airport four hours early. "I'm afraid they'll hand her to me and she'll start crying and cry for the next eighteen years!" Robin fretted.

"There'll be operating instructions for her from the foster mom, right?" Larry whispered. He never got an answer. Instead, he got a daughter. Bright-eyed and alert, thirteen pounds and a week shy of six months old. Mackenzie was delivered into her parents' arms — without a peep — by the retired cop who'd escorted her since Los Angeles.

It was a special delivery, indeed.

Marli Murphy
The Kansas City Star, 1998

Afterward

New parenthood does the funniest things to normal people, doesn't it? How nice to share with each other, the trials and tribulations of our special memories, and revel in the wonder of our journey into parenthood.

If you have a favorite, true story from pregnancy, childbirth, adoption or new parenthood you'd like to share — send it to us. "Stork Search" is looking for you!

Please see next page for details or visit our website at: **www.bellylaughs.com**

Our deepest thanks to all the wonderful parents and grandparents who have shared, and continue to share, their legacies of love and laughter. We are proud to donate all profits from *Belly Laughs and Babies* to parent/baby charitable programs.

Long live parenthood fun!

You are Invited to Share the Fun at a

Belly Laughs & Babies'
Baby Shower!

At: Stork Search
P.O. Box 860700
Shawnee Mission, KS 66286

Up to $1,000 in Cash Prizes

Due Date: Delivery of your story and entry form to *Belly Laughs and Babies* makes you a contestant. Cash prizes awarded! If you go past the due date, send your story anyway — we hope to give birth to a new *Belly Laughs & Babies* book soon! Stories must be true and unpublished, 750 words or less.

Given by: Laughing Stork Press

Registered at: www.bellylaughs.com

Check in regularly for updates and due dates! Or send a S.A.S.E. to the above mailing address and we'll send you a form.

Special Requests: Invite your friends, family, one and all, to shower us with baby anecdotes and escapades from pregnancy to new parenthood. Check details at: www.bellylaughs.com

RSVP: mary@bellylaughs.com
Fax: 913-422-7988

Remember, the fun starts when your story makes its grand entrance!

Contributor's Index

Anslinger, B.	p. 90		Harm, L.	p. 169
Bader Jones, J.	p. 81		Harvey, M.	p. 72
Barnes, M.	p. 132		Hayes, S.	p. 153
Berry, T.	p. 128		Hayes, T.	p. 56
Brandeis, G.	p. 29		Hinson, K.	p. 128
Breese, S.	p. 70		Hoey, M.	p. 18
Breese, S.	p. 26		Hopkins, M.	p. 60
Breslin, S.	p. 96		Hoover, S.	p. 6
Brown, D.	p. 50		Houston, G.	p. 16
Bryant, G.	p. 31		Huston, D.	p. 171
Bundridge, W.	p. 101		Inga	p. 89
Choate, J.	p. 83		James, F.	p. 107
Colson, W.	p. 64		Janicke, P.	p. 93
Colson, W.	p. 153		Jenks, L.	p. 143
Corcoran, L.	p. 135		Jewell, B.	p. 156
Crisman, M.	p. 7		Kamberg, M.	p. 17
Daarud, C.	p. 152		Kamberg, M.	p. 120
D'Alessandro	p. 179		Katz, C.	p. 38
Davidson, W.	p. 8		Katz, C.	p. 78
Davidson, W.	p. 130		Kelly, K.	p. 51
Dolan, N.	p. 41		Kite, P.	p. 196
Eckels, M.	p. 107		Klenetsky, W.	p. 121
Ficka, W.	p. 137		Kobylinski, R.	p. 112
Fred, V.	p. 171		Krantz, K.	p. 63
Freund, C.	p. 111		Lauer, L.	p. 22
Gall, J.	p. 46		Linderer, D.	p. 5
Garitano, R.	p. 113		Litt, J.	p. 195
Genell, J.	p. 49		Lopata, P.	p. 200
Ghesquierre, D.	p. 77		Mazer, J.	p. 8
Grafke, N.	p. 162		McAllister, E.	p. 91

Contributor's Index (cont'd.)

McDonough	p. 63	Rudolph, B.	p. 150
McKelvey, T.	p. 147	Schindorff, D.	p. 25
Mesenbrink, S.	p. 39	Schirmer, J.	p. 186
Michna, E.	p. 132	Schuckel, K.	p. 61
Miller, V.	p. 108	Shine, M.	p. 154
Morgan, M.	p. 59	Shine, M.	p. 155
Morris, C.	p. 42	Shine, M.	p. 157
Mueller, D.	p. 152	Shirley, B.	p. 158
Murphy, C.	p. 15	Sloan, T.	p. 134
Murphy, M.	p. 98	Smith, F.	p. 110
Murphy, M.	p. 205	Smith, P.	p. 86
Myers, N.	p. 77	Summerlin, S.	p. 62
Norwood, I.	p. 121	Sutton, J.	p. 164
Norwood, I.	p. 135	Sykes, Melissa	p. 48
O'Brien, D.	p. 116	Vernon, M.	p. 161
Oliver, E.	p. 67	Wallace, R.	p. 119
Pacey, A.	p. 7	Webb, T.	p. 23
Park, S.	p. 4	Webb, T.	p. 65
Perdew, L.	p. 173	Weldon, M.	p. 33
Potts, B.	p. 36	Weldon, M.	p. 36
Purl, A.	p. 109	Welch, L.	p. 64
Powis, J.	p. 43	Whitaker, P.	p. 115
Rabas, J.	p. 177	Zari, R.	p. 115
Rachkus Uttich	p. 12		
Robinson, A.	p. 127		

Mary Sheridan

Mary, sentimental at heart, loves to hear tales of parenthood. Watching birth re-enactments on television, or at the movies, never leaves her with a dry eye. Married to an obstetrician/gynecologist for nearly 20 years, she has gleaned many personal "stork" experiences from those nightly phone interruptions to a good night's sleep. With three children in tow, ages 15, 12, and 9, real-life experience adds to the fun!

Professional medical experience includes eight years in a university hospital as a nuclear medicine technologist and working as a clinical office nurse in her husband's OB/GYN practice. Since having children, professional time has mainly been spent in real estate property management.

As a true, community servant at heart, she has worn many volunteer hats. From PTA school activities to president of her Junior League and president of her county's volunteer-based health clinic for the medically indigent, her commitment to the community stands. For the past four years, she has also served as a planning commissioner for her city.

Her "top" hat now is acquiring and sharing the "untold" stories of some of the most remarkable people on earth — PARENTS!

Melissa Muldoon

Melissa is an illustrator, graphic designer and dedicated mom. She balances work with raising three energetic little boys, ages 9, 6 and 1 year.

Belly Laughs & Babies' Hall of Fame

Virginia Mandacina

Joanne Barrett

Susan Gitlin

Kathleen Stander

Penny Silvers

Lori Slagle

Becky Walker

Susan Everett

Marjorie Hopkins

Florence Smith

Michele Weldon

Sally Breslin

Jeffrey Gall

Kathleen Kelly

Pat Kite

Mary Jane Vernon

Toni Webb

Twyla Hayes

Jim Schirmer

Julie Mazer

We would love to add your name to our list. Take a moment to share your family's special story. Enter the Stork Search contest today. You, too, could be a winner! Visit us at: **www.bellylaughs.com**

Available at Bookstores or Order a Copy of
Belly Laughs and Babies
by Fax, Phone, E-mail or U.S. Post

FAX Orders: (913-422-7988)

Telephone Orders: Call Toll Free: 1-888-895-BABY

E-mail: www.bellylaughs.com

U.S. Post: Laughing Stork Press, P.O. Box 860700
Shawnee Mission, KS 66286, U.S.A
(Send the order form below with check, or credit card information)

_____ Number of copies Of **Belly Laughs and Babies** at $9.95
(Sales Tax included)

_____ SUBTOTAL (Quantity x $9.95)

_____ Number of copies Of **Belly Laughs and Babies 2** at $10.95
(Sales Tax included)

_____ SUBTOTAL (Quantity x $10.95)

_____ Priority Shipping (USA only: $3.00 postage 1-4 books)

_____ **TOTAL DUE**

Name: _____

Company: _____

Address: _____

City: _____

State: _____ **Zip:** _____

Telephone: (_____) _____

☐ Check ☐ Credit Card ☐ *VISA* ☐ *MasterCard* ☐ *Discover*

Card Number: _____

Name on Card: _____

Exp. Date: _____

Signature: _____

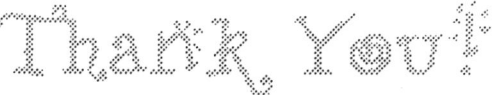